Medical Imaging in Gastroenterology and Hepatology

FALK SYMPOSIUM 124

Medical Imaging in Gastroenterology and Hepatology

Edited by

F. Hagenmüller
*Innere Medizin I
Allgemeines Krankenhaus Altona
Hamburg
Germany*

M. P. Manns
*Gastroenterologie/Hepatologie
Medizinische Hochschule
Hannover
Hannover
Germany*

H.-G. Musmann
*Institut für Theoretische
Nachrichtentechnik
TU Hannover
Hannover
Germany*

J. F. Riemann
*Gastroenterologie/Hepatologie
Klinikum der Stadt Ludwigshafen
Ludwigshafen
Germany*

Proceedings of Falk Symposium 124 (Progress in Gastroenterology and Hepatology Part I) held in Hannover, Germany, September 28–29, 2001

KLUWER ACADEMIC PUBLISHERS
DORDRECHT / BOSTON / LONDON

Library of Congress Cataloging-in-Publication Data is available.

ISBN 0-7923-8774-0

Published by Kluwer Academic Publishers, BV
P.O. Box 17, 3300 AA Dordrecht, The Netherlands.

Sold and distributed in North, Central and South America
by Kluwer Academic Publishers,
101 Philip Drive, Norwell, MA 02061, USA.

In all other countries, sold and distributed
by Kluwer Academic Publishers, Distribution Center,
P.O. Box 322, 3300 AH Dordrecht, The Netherlands.

Printed on acid-free paper

All rights reserved
© 2002 Kluwer Academic Publishers and Falk Foundation e.V.

No part of the material protected by this copyright notice may be reproduced or utilized in any form or by any means, electronic or mechanical, including photocopying, recording or by any information storage and retrieval system, without written prior permission from the copyright owners.

Printed and bound in Great Britain by MPG Books, Bodmin, Cornwall.

Contents

List of principal contributors   viii

Section I: PROJECTS AND PERSPECTIVES

1. Cortical imaging of visceral function and disease   3
P Enck, H Hinninghofen and B Wietek

2. Minilaparoscopy – a new diagnostic tool   13
J M Zeeh, U Treichel and G Gerken

3. Laparoscopy and endoscopy – competitive or complementary?   21
H Feussner and E Frimberger

Section II: IMAGE AND EVIDENCE

4. Chronic pancreatitis: an evident role for endoscopy   33
J Devière and J-M Dumonceau

5. Endosonography – what are the diagnostic advantages?   40
R H Hawes

Section III: PROCEDURE AND PERCEPTION

6. What is the time required for a good endoscopy?
Time for training   53
G A Lehman

7. Improved gastrointestinal imaging – improved outcome for the patients?   55
S Hollerbach

CONTENTS

8	What does the surgeon expect from preoperative imaging in liver tumours? T Becker, H S B Frericks, F Lehner, R Lück, H Bektas, B Nashan, M Galanski and J Klempnauer	69

Section IV: CO-EXISTENCE OF IMAGING TECHNIQUES

9	Scintigraphy/positron emission tomography (PET) – complementary support for endoscopy W H Knapp, K F Gratz and A R Börner	79
10	Magnetic resonance imaging: a substitute for endoscopy? H E Adamek, J Albert, H Breer and J F Riemann	90
11	Three-dimensional (3D) imaging: from sectional image to 3D model M A Barish	94

Section V: NETWORK SYSTEMS

12	Training models – why and how? S Bar-Meir	109
13	The Minimal Standard Terminology for digestive endoscopy: introduction to structured reporting M Delvaux	112

Section VI: ULTRASOUND

14	Ultrasound in diffuse liver disease L Bolondi, S Gaiani, N Celli and F Piscaglia	127
15	Use of ultrasound contrast agents in hepatology A K P Lim, C J Harvey, S D Taylor-Robinson, M J K Blomley and D O Cosgrove	132
16	Percutaneous interventional therapy of liver cancer T Livraghi	140
17	Clinical role of ultrasound in biliary disease S Wagner	151
18	Diagnostic approach to unclear liver tumours J Schölmerich	158

Section VII: IMAGING – NEW TECHNOLOGIES

19	Fluorescence endoscopy in gastroenterology H Messmann and E Endlicher	173

20	Chromoendoscopy *M I F Canto*	182
21	CT- or MRI-based virtual colonography *A G Schreyer and H Herfarth*	194
22	Three-dimensional endoscopy *T Thormählen, H Broszio and P N Meier*	199

Section VIII: NEW ENDOSCOPIC EQUIPMENT – NEW VISUAL PERSPECTIVES?

23	Wireless capsule endoscopy *A Glukhovsky and H Jacob*	215
24	When is enteroscopy useful? *G Gay*	225
25	Focal point: oesophago-cardial transition *H W Boyce*	226
	Index	229

List of Principal Contributors

H E Adamek
Klinikum der Stadt Ludwigshafen
Innere Medizin C
Bremserstr. 79
D-67063 Ludwigshafen
Germany

S Bar-Meir
Chaim Sheba Medical Center
Department of Gastroenterology
52 621 Tel Hashomer
Israel

M A Barish
Boston Medical Center
Boston University School of Medicine
Boston, MA 02118
USA

T Becker
Klinik für Viszeral- und
 Transplantationschirurgie
Medizinische Hochschule Hannover
Carl-Neuberg-Str. 1
D-30625 Hannover
Germany

L Bolondi
Università di Bologna
Policlinico S. Orsola-Malpighi
Dip. Med. Interna e
 Gastroenterologia
Via Albertoni 15
I-40138 Bologna
Italy

M I F Canto
Division of Therapeutic Endoscopy
 and Endoscopic Ultrasonography
The Johns Hopkins University School
 of Medicine
1830 Monument Street,
Room 425
Baltimore, Maryland 21205
USA

M Delvaux
CHU Rangueil
Gastroenterology Unit
F-31403 Toulouse Cedex 04
France

J Devière
ULB – Hôpital Erasme
Department of Gastroenterology
Route de Lennik 808
B-1070 Bruxelles
Belgium

P Enck
Universitätsklinikum Tübingen
Allgemeine Chirurgie – Victor von
 Bruns Laboratorien
Waldhörnlestr. 22
D-72072 Tübingen
Germany

H Feussner
Chirurgische Klinik und Poliklinik
Technische Universität
Klinikum Rechts der Isar
Ismaninger Str. 22
D-81675 München
Germany

G Gay
Service de Médicine Interne
Hôpital de Brabois
Allée du Morvan
F-54511 Vandœvre-Lés-Nancy Cedex
France

LIST OF PRINCIPAL CONTRIBUTORS

G Gerken
Gastroenterologie/Hepatologie
Universitätsklinikum
Hufelandstr. 55
D-45147 Essen
Germany

A Glukhovsky
Given Imaging Ltd.
New Industrial Park
PO Box 258
Yoqneam 20692
Israel

F Hagenmüller
Innere Medizin I
Allgemeines Krankenhaus Altona
Paul-Ehrlich-Str. 1
D-22763 Hamburg
Germany

R H Hawes
Medical University of South Carolina
Digestive Disease Center
96 Jonathan Lucas Street,
Ste 210 CSB
Charleston, SC 29425
USA

H Herfarth
Innere Medizin I
Klinikum der Universität
 Regensburg
D-93042 Regensburg
Germany

S Hollerbach
Ruhr-Universität Medizinische
 Univ.-Klinik
Knappschaftskrankenhaus
In der Schornau 23–25
D-44892 Bochum
Germany

W H Knapp
Abteilung Nuklearmedizin
Medizinische Hochschule
 Hannover
Carl-Neuberg-Str. 1
D-30625 Hannover
Germany

G A Lehman
Division of Gastroenterology &
 Hepatology
University Hospital
550 N. University Blvd., Rm. 2300
Indianapolis, Indiana 4602-5000
USA

A K P Lim
Robert Steiner MRI Unit
Hammersmith Hospital
Du Cane Road
London, W12 0NN
UK

T Livraghi
Ospedale Civile di Vimercate
Divisione di Radiologia
Via Cesare Battisti 23
I-20059 Vimercate
Italy

M P Manns
Gastroenterologie/Hepatologie
Medizinische Hochschule
 Hannover
Carl-Neuberg-Str. 1
D-30625 Hannover
Germany

H Messmann
III Medizinische Klinik
Klinikum Augsburg
D-86009 Augsburg
Germany

H-G Musmann
Institut für Theoretische
 Nachrichtentechnik
TU Hannover
Schneiderberg 32
D-30167 Hannover
Germany

J F Riemann
Gastroenterologie/Hepatologie
Klinikum der Stadt Ludwigshafen
Bremserstr. 79
D-67063 Ludwigshafen
Germany

J Schölmerich
Innere Medizin I
Klinikum der Universität
 Regensburg
D-93042 Regensburg
Germany

A G Schreyer
Department of Radiology
University Hospital Regensburg
Franz-Josef-Strauss Allee 11
D-93053 Regensburg
Germany

LIST OF PRINCIPAL CONTRIBUTORS

T Thormählen
Institut für Theoretische
 Nachrichtentechnik
TU Hannover
Schneiderberg 32
D-30167 Hannover
Germany

S Wagner
Medizinische Klinik II
Klinikum Deggendorf
D-94469 Deggendorf
Germany

H Worth Boyce
University School of Florida
Section of Gastroenterology
Medical Center – Box 19
12901 Bruce B Downs Blvd.
Tampa, FL 33612
USA

Section I
Projects and perspectives

1
Cortical imaging of visceral function and disease

P. ENCK, H. HINNINGHOFEN and B. WIETEK

CORTICAL EVOKED POTENTIALS FOLLOWING INTESTINAL STIMULATION

More than 10 years ago, Frieling and co-workers[1,2] for the first time attempted to solve the question of how visceral sensations are delivered to and processed by the brain, by using neurophysiological tools such as evoked potential (EP) recordings to directly investigate the human gut–brain axis. This had previously been done only for the human bladder[3]. Within a few years studies all over the world had demonstrated that EP recordings may be used to assess the basic mechanisms and rules of the gut–brain pathway and their integrity, not only in healthy subjects but also in patients with various intestinal and extraintestinal disorders (see below). This work has been summarized by Enck and Frieling[4] and others[5,6]. Intestinal EPs were recorded not only following electrical or mechanical (balloon) stimulation but also with chemical stimuli applied to oesophageal mucosa[7]; other intestinal compartments such as the stomach or the small intestine were not studied, due to methodological difficulties applying these stimuli in a reliable and safe way. A single study recorded cortical EP following shockwave treatment of the gallbladder with various lithotripters, but from the data reported it remains unclear as to whether somatosensory or visceral EPs were recorded[8].

Comparing EPs from the viscera with those of the body's periphery made clear that both similarities and differences account for the specifics of visceral perception. For example, EPs from the oesophagus and rectum are usually much longer in latency and smaller in amplitude than somatosensory EPs, and they decrease in size with increasing stimulation frequency (above 1 Hz) and duration; however, they correlate positively with the stimulation intensity, as do somatosensory EPs[9,10]. This explains to some extent their specific psychophysiological characteristics. It was also made clear that EPs from the oesophagus are transmitted via the vagal nerve, since direct vagal stimulation using a pacemaker produced similar brain responses[11]. However, the relative contribution of spinal pathways to cortical EP following (painful) stimulation remains an open question, since spinal primary and secondary sensitization has been shown to occur following oesophageal acid exposure[12].

With EP recordings, e.g. from the oesophagus, it was also possible to identify differences in the innervation of the proximal and distal part, as the two were different in their shape and latency, but any further description of their cortical representation was obsolete. It became evident quite early that using EP technology would not allow precise localization of the cortical regions in which visceral afferent data are processed[13]; the reason for this limitation of EP recordings is the fact that an electrical field generated by one or more brain dipoles is comparably large (e.g. compared to the magnetic fields, see the next section), which inversely allows only a raw estimate of the dipole numbers and their localization when an electrical field is recorded by multichannel EP. However, some of the brain mapping work published already identified relevant cortical areas involved in the processing of visceral afferent sensations, e.g. the insular cortex. Any further question, e.g. that of topographic organization of different intestinal compartments (lower and upper oesophagus, for instance), could also not be answered with EP recordings.

Consequently only a few EP studies were performed in patients, e.g. with autonomic neuropathy due to diabetes[14], with chest pain of cardiac and non-cardiac origin[15–18], spinal cord injury[19], constipation[20] and dyspepsia[21]. Results were inconsistent with respect to any specificity of EP responses compared to healthy controls; e.g. in patients with diabetic autonomic neuropathy no EPs rather than altered EP responses were observed; this limits its potential use in clinical diagnosis. In chest-pain patients, the only group which has been studied repetitively by independent researchers, it was consistently shown that EPs were reduced in amplitude in patients when compared to healthy control subjects, indicating changes in processing at a central level, rather than at peripheral receptor level, to be responsible for pathological perception of visceral sensation.

The focus on functional bowel disorders and their assumed sensory pathomechanisms (visceral hypersensitivity and hyperalgesia etc., see the first section) called for further evaluation of differences in central processing of visceral afferent, to which EP recordings can contribute only if the cortical areas of interest are known and agreed; this is not yet the case.

BRAIN MAPPING OF INTESTINAL SENSORY FUNCTIONS

With wider availability of brain imaging technology, especially positron emission tomography (PET), functional magnetic resonance imaging (fMRI), magnetoencephalography (MEG), and single-photon emission tomography (SPECT), it was a matter of time until the first utilization of these techniques was reported for intestinal functions. A PET study during oesophageal stimulation[22] marked the beginning of a series of papers using these techniques for the upper and lower gastrointestinal compartment (Tables 1 and 2), both in control subjects and in patients; they were recently reviewed by Aziz and Thompson[23] and Aziz et al.[24]. For technical details of these methods the reader is referred to these reviews.

Table 1 Brain imaging studies following oesophaegal stimulation in healthy controls

Main author	Year	Ref.	Technique	Design	Stimulus	Intensity	Position	Controls
Aziz	1997	22	PET	(Block)	Balloon	No-pain–pain	Distal	$n = 8$
Kern	1998	25	fMRI	Block	Acid–balloon	Below pain	Distal	$n = 10$
Binkofski	1998	26	fMRI	Block	Balloon	No-pain–pain	Distal	$n = 5$
Furlong	1998	27	MEG	ER	Balloon	Below pain	Prox–distal	$n = 34$
Schnitzler	1999	28	MEG	ER	Electrical	Below pain	Distal	$n = 7$
Loose	1999	29	MEG	ER	Balloon	No-pain–pain	Prox–distal	$n = 6$
Hecht	1999	30	MEG	ER	Electrical	Below pain	Prox–distal	$n = 9$
Aziz	2000	31	fMRI	Block	Balloon	Below pain	Prox–distal	$n = 6$

Parenthesis indicate non-significant activation to some

Table 2 Brain imaging studies following anorectal stimulation

Main author	Year	Ref.	Technique	Design	Anal	Rectum	Controls	Patients
Silverman	1997	32	PET	(Block)	No	Balloon	$n = 6$	$n = 6$
Baciu	1999	33	fMRI	Block	No	Balloon	$n = 8$	—
Bouras	1999	34	SPECT	(Block)	No	Balloon	$n = 10$	—
Mertz	2000	35	fMRI	Block	No	Balloon	$n = 16$	$n = 18$
Stottrop	2000	36	MEG	E-R	Electrical	No	$n = 7$	—
Hobday	2001	37	fMRI	Block	No	Balloon	$n = 8$	—
Binkofski	2001	38	fMRI	Block	Electrical	Electrical	$n = 8$	—
Lotze	2001	38	fMRI	E-R	Balloon	Balloon	$n = 8$	—
Kern	2000	40	fMRI	Block	No	Balloon	$n = 8$	—
Nabiloff	2000	41	PET	(Block)	No	Balloon	$n = 12$	$n = 12$
Ringel	2000	42	PET	(Block)	No	Balloon	$n = 6$	$n = 6$
Bonaz	2000	43	fMRI	Block	No	Balloon	—	$n = 8$

Parentheses indicate non-significant activation to some

It is evident from this work that different technologies have advantages and limitations in elucidating brain processing of visceral afferents information. For example, with a block design in fMRI (and also in PET studies) all information on the time sequence of areas activated is lost, while event-related processing of data – as is regularily done with electrophysiological methods (EP, MEG) but has recently also been applied to fMRI – temporal resolution is much better.

Among the first questions addressed was whether intestinal compartments are represented over the primary sensory (S1) cortex – better known as the 'homunculus' – in humans. Since PET and fMRI do not provide much information regarding the timing of cortical events, this could be answered only using MEG, which has a high temporal resolution. It was shown[28,29] that cortical responses from the upper and lower oesophagus – in contrast to somatosensory afferents – are directly projected onto the second somatosensory (S2) cortex (Figure 1), but share some of the psychophysiological characteristics of primary somatosensory (S1) responses; a somatotopy of the S2 cortex has so far not been identified. This may explain the rather diffuse character of visceral, intestinal sensations with respect to localization.

Different from the oesophagus, the anal canal has been shown to activate somatosensory and visceral pathways since it is represented both over the S1 cortext – halfway inbetween the hand and foot representation – as well as over

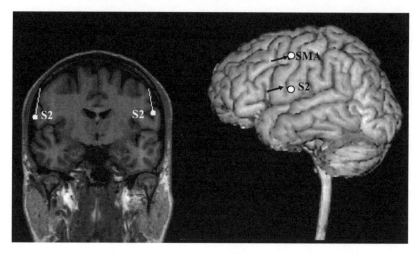

Figure 1 Magnetoencephalographic response (MEG dipoles projected onto an individual brain anatomy) after electrical stimulation of the lower oesophagus. The early response is located bilaterally in the S2 cortex, the late response in the supplementary motor cortex (SMA) (from ref. 29)

the S2 cortex[36] (Figure 2); this is unique in comparison to any other intestinal section imaged so far.

Electrophysiological tools such as MEG are limited to detecting activity at the cortical surface only; any brain activity below 2 cm from the surface requires other technology. It is, however, clear that most relevant processing of visceral information is occurring at deeper brain structures such as the midbrain and brainstem. Consequently, the work of the most recent years has focused on identifying the entire brain network of lower gastrointestinal functions using PET and fMRI.

From published papers and abstracts the 'anorectal brain network' identified so far is summarized in Table 3. It includes, besides the S1 and S2 cortices, the insular cortex (IN), the anterior cingulate gyrus (CG), the prefrontal cortex (PFC), the thalamus (Th), and the parieto-orbital cortex (POC); in single studies, activations of the supplementary motor cortex (SMA, for anal stimulation), the hippocampus, brainstem (periaqueductal grey, medulla), and cerebellum (for anal but not for rectal stimulation) were observed (Figure 3).

It is obvious from the complexity of the network that most of these activated areas cannot serve specific intestinal functions, but share responsibility with other afferent processes; e.g. pain processing irrespective of its origin is known to involve different sections of the CG depending on whether pain intensity or pain quality is affected[44]. The PFC is engaged in vigilance and attention[45], the POC is activated with interference of body image[46], and the limbic circuitry (hypothalamus, hippocampus, ACG) is a central network for processing of emotions in general.

As with EP recordings, brain imaging of visceral functions was immediately used for identifying central pathomechanisms in patients with functional bowel disorders, after a first study by Silverman *et al.*[32] had shown a lacking correlation of ACG activation with perceived stimulus intensity (rectal balloon distension) in irritable bowel syndrome (IBS) patients as compared to healthy controls; in

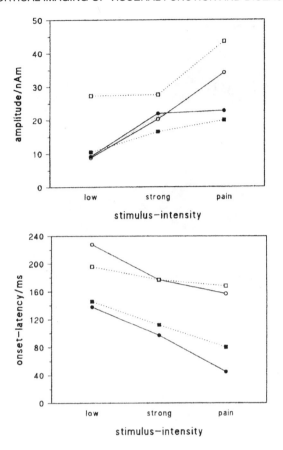

Figure 2 Psychophysiological characteristics of MEG responses in the S2 cortex following electrical oesophageal stimulation with different intensities. Note the decrease in the latency (below) and increase in amplitude (above) with increasing stimulus intensity (from ref. 29)

contrast, IBS patients showed more PFC activation than their counterparts. The authors concluded that a central mechanism of decreased descending inhibition of pain pathways is responsible for visceral hyperalgesia in IBS. However, this may be a premature conclusion since other studies (e.g. ref. 35) could not confirm this central difference in pain processing between IBS and normals, but described in part other alteration. A clear association of quantitative brain activation with the psychophysiological characteristics of visceral stimuli has not yet been shown, either in healthy subjects or in patients. A first study in patients undergoing rectal resection and pouch surgery has recently extended applications into the question of neural plasticity at the cortical level[47], and one of the most promising possibilities will include changes in brain activation biofeedback after biofeedback training.

While the sensory anorectal brain network seems well established, much work needs to be done on the other intestinal functions and compartments.

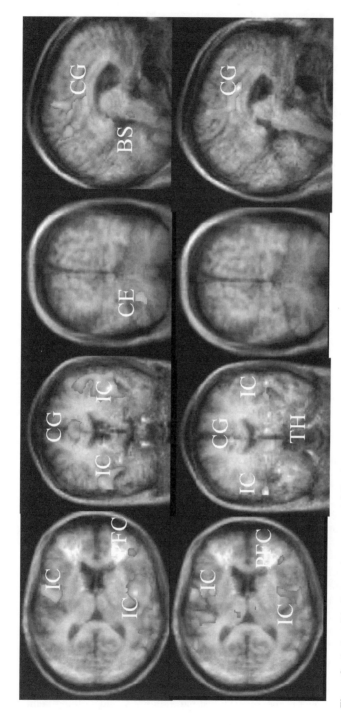

Figure 3 Activated brain areas (group means) following anal (top row) and rectal (bottom row) mechanical stimulation as recorded with event-related functional MRI. The sections show the insular cortex (IC) and the cingulate gyrus (CG), the prefrontal cortex (PFC), the cerebellum (CE), the brainstem (BS) and the orbitoparietal cortex (OPC) (from ref. 38)

Table 3 The anorectal brain network according to published studies

Main author	Year	Ref.	S1–S2	Ins	ACG	CG	PFC	Th	AM	CE	OPC	BS
Silverman	1997	32			×	(×)	×				(×)	
Baciu	1999	33		×	×	×	×				×	
Bouras	1999	34			×		×	×				
Mertz	2000	35		×	×		×	×				×
Stottrop	2000	36	×									
Binkofski	2000	37	×	×	×	×	×			×		×
Lotze	2000	38	×	×	×	×	×	(×)	(×)	(×)	×	(×)
Hobday	2001	39	×	×	×	×	×					
Kern	2000	40	(×)		×		×	×				
Nabiloff	2000	41		×	×	×	×	×	×		×	
Ringel	2000	42			×							
Bonaz	2000	43		×	×		×				×	

Parentheses indicate non-significant activation to some extent.

S1, S2 : primary and secondary sensory cortex
Ins : insular cortex
ACG : Anterior cingulate gyrus
CG : Cingulate gyrus
PFC : Prefrontal cortex
Th : Thalamus
AM : Amygdala
CE : Cerebellum
OPC : Operculum
BS : Brain stem

Investigation of motor functions of the anorectum are still at an early stage[48], but neccessary to fully understand mechanisms of defaecation and continence; investigation of cortical representation of micturition in health and disease could serve as a recently established example[49]. For the oesophagus, cortical representation of motor functions during swallowing using this and other technology (e.g. motor evoked potential – MEP – recording) have been shown to be of help, e.g. understanding dysphagia in stroke[50], and experimental manipulation of cortical processing of visceral afferents by emotions and other central 'states' may help to explain functional gastrointestinal disorders[51,52]. First data are available following stimulation of the stomach[53] and this will soon allow cortical imaging during nausea development[54]. Furthermore, fMRI studies during eating[55] have shown that, with imaging technology, cortical metabolic processes can be investigated. Finally, PET studies identifying serotonin and histamine receptor binding in the human brain during rectal stimulation[56,57], and medical treatment with a 5-HT-3 antagonist (alosetron) has been shown to alter the response of the brain with balloon distension, especially in the limbic circuitry[58].

References

1. Frieling T, Enck P, Wienbeck M. Cerebral responses evoked by electrical stimulation of rectosigmoid in normal subjects. Dig Dis Sci. 1989;34:202–5.
2. Frieling T, Enck P, Wienbeck M. Cerebral responses evoked by electrical stimulation of the esophagus in normal subjects. Gastroenterology. 1989;97:475–8.

3. Badr G, Carlsson CA, Fall M, Friberg S, Lindström L, Ohlsson B. Cortical evoked potentials following stimulation of the urinary bladder in man. Electroenceph Clin Neurophysiol. 1982;54:494–8.
4. Enck P, Frieling T. Human gut–brain interactions. J Gastrointest Motil. 1993;5:77–87.
5. Hollerbach S, Tougas G, Frieling T et al. Cerebral evoked potentials (EP) following electrical and mechanical stimulation of visceral organs in humans. Crit Rev Biomed Eng. 1997; 25:203–42.
6. Aziz Q, Thompson DG. Brain gut axis in health and disease. Gastroenterology. 1998;114: 559–78.
7. Roscher S, Renner B, Kuhlbusch R, Frieling T, Kobal G, Enck P. Cerebral activation after chemical and mechanical stimulation of the esophagus. Gastroenterology. 1998;114:A168.
8. Schneider TC, Hummel T, Janowitz P et al. Pain in extracorporeal shock-wave lithotripsy: a comparison of different lithotripsers in volunteers. Gastroenterology. 1992;102:640–6.
9. Söllenböhmer C, Enck P, Häussinger D, Frieling T. Electrically evoked cerebral potentials during esophageal distension at perception and pain threshold. Am J Gastroenterol. 1996;91:970–5.
10. Hollerbach S, Kamath MV, Chen Y, Fitzpatrick D, Upton ARM, Tougas G. The magnitude of the central response to esophageal electrical stimulation is intensity dependent. Gastroenterology. 1997;112:1137–46.
11. Tougas G, Hudoba P, Fitzpatrick D, Hunt RH, Upton ARM. Cerebral evoked responses following direct vagal and esophageal electrical stimulation in humans. Am J Physiol. 1993;264:G486–91.
12. Sarkar S, Hobson A, Woolf CJ et al. Oesophageal cortical evoked potentials are potentiated following acid induced hypersensitivity. Gut. 1999;44:(Suppl. 1):A111.
13. Aziz Q, Furlong PL, Barlow J et al. Topographic mapping of cortical potentials evoked by distension of the human proximal and distal oesophagus. Electroenceph Clin Neurophysiol. 1995;96:219–28.
14. Rathmann W, Enck P, Frieling T, Gries FA. Visceral afferent neuropathy in diabetic gastroparesis. Diabetes Care. 1991;14:1086–9.
15. Smout AJP, DeVore MS, Dalton CB, Castell DO. Cerebral potentials evoked by oesophageal distension in patients with non-cardiac chest pain. Gut. 1992;33:298–302.
16. Frobert O, Arendt-Nielsen L, Bak P, Funch-Jensen P, Bagger JP. Pain perception and brain evoked potentials in patients with angina despite nomal coronary angiograms. Heart. 1995;75:436–41.
17. DeVault KR, Castell DO. Esophageal balloon distention and cerebral evoked potential recording in the evaluation of unexplained chest pain. Am J Med. 1992;92:20–6.
18. Hollerbach ST, Bulat R, May A et al. Abnormal cerebral processing of oesophageal stimuli in patients with noncardiac chest pain. Neurogastroenterology. 2000;12:555–66.
19. DeVault KR, Beacham S, Castell DO, Streletz LJ, Ditunno JF. Esophageal sensation in spinal cord-injured patients: balloon distension and cerebral evoked potential recording. Am J Physiol. 1996;271:G937–41.
20. Loening-Baucke V, Yamada T. Is the afferent pathway from the rectum impaired in children with chronic constipation and encopresis? Gastroenterology. 1995;109:397–403.
21. Kanazawa M, Nomura T, Fukodo S, Hono M. Abnormal visceral perception in patients with functional dyspepsia: use of cerebral potentials by electrical stimulation of the esophagus. Neurogastroenterology. 2000;12:87–94.
22. Aziz Q, Andersson J, Valind S et al. Identification of the brain loci processing human oesophageal sensation using positron emission tomography. Gastroenterology. 1997;113:50–9.
23. Aziz Q, Thompson DG. Brain–gut axis in health and disease. Gastroenterology. 1998; 114:559–78.
24. Aziz Q, Schnitzler A, Enck P. Functional neuro-imaging of visceral sensation. J Clin Neurophysiol. 2000;17:604–12.
25. Kern MK, Birn RM, Jaradeh S et al. Identification and characterization of cerebral cortical response to esophageal mucosal acid exposure and distention. Gastroenterology. 1998; 115: 1353–62.
26. Binkofski F, Schnitzler A, Enck P et al. Somatic and limbic cortex activation in esophageal distension: a functional magnetic resonance imaging study. Ann Neurol. 1998;44:811–15.
27. Furlong PL, Aziz Q, Singh KD, Thompson DG, Hobson A, Harding GF. Cortical localization of magnetic fields evoked by esophageal distension. Electroenceph Clin Neurophysiol. 1998; 108:234–43.

28. Schnitzler A, Volkmann J, Enck P, Frieling T, Witte OW, Freund HJ. Differential cortical organization of visceral and somatic sensation in humans: a neuromagnetic study. Eur J Neurosci. 1999;11:305–15.
29. Loose R, Schnitzler A, Sarkar S et al. Cortical activation during mechanical esophageal stimulation: a neuromagnetic study. Neurogastroenterology. 1999;11:163–71.
30. Hecht M, Kober H, Claus D, Hilz M, Vieth J, Neundörfer B. The electrical and magnetic cerebral responses evoked by electrical stimulation of the esophagus and the location of their cerebral sources. Electroenceph Clin Neurophysiol. 1999;110:1435–44.
31. Aziz Q, Thompson DG, Ng VWK et al. Cortical processing of human somatic and visceral sensation. J Neurosci. 2000;20:2657–63.
32. Silverman DHS, Munakata JA, Ennes H, Madelkern MA, Hon CK, Mayer EA. Regional cerebral activity in normal and pathological perception of visceral pain. Gastroenterology. 1997;112:64–72.
33. Baciu MV, Bonaz BL, Papillon EP et al. Central processing of rectal pain: a functional MRI imaging study. Am J Neuroradiol. 1999;20:1920–4.
34. Bouras EP, O'Brien TJ, Camilleri M, O'Connor MK, Mullan BP. Cerebral topography of rectal stimulation using single photon emission computed tomography. Am J Physiol. 1999;227:G687–94.
35. Mertz H, Morgan V, Tanner G et al. Regional cerebral activation in irritable bowel syndrome and control subjects with painful and nonpainful rectal distention. Gastroenterology. 2000;118:842–8.
36. Stottrop K, Schnitzler A, Witte OW, Freund HJ, Enck P. Cortical representation of the anal canal. Gastroenterology. 1998;114:A167.
37. Binkofski F, Schnitzler A, Stottrop K, Enck P. Cortical representation of anal and rectal sensation. A fMRI-study. J Neurophysiol. 2001;14:1027–34.
38. Lotze M, Wietek B, Birbaumer N, Ehrhardt J, Grodd W, Enck P. Cerebral activation during anal and rectal stimulation. NeuroImage. 2001;14:1027–34.
39. Hobday DI, Aziz Q, Thacker N, Hollander I, Jackson A, Thompson DG. A study of the cortical processing of ano-rectal sensitization using functional MRI. Brain. 2001;124:361–8.
40. Kern MK, Arndorfer RC, Shaker R. Effects of effort on cerebral cortical activity during volitional external anal sphincter contraction. Gastroenterology. 2000;118:A445.
41. Nabiloff BD, Derbyshire SW, Munaka J et al. Evidence for decreased activation of central fear circuits by expected adversive visceral stimuli in IBS patients. Gastroenterology. 2000;118:A137.
42. Ringel Y, Drossman DA, Turkington TG et al. Dysfunction of the motivational–affective pain system in patients with IBS: PET brain imaging in response to rectal balloon distension. Gastroenterology. 2000;118:A444.
43. Bonaz BL, Papillon E, Baciu M et al. Central processing of rectal pain in IBS patients: an fMRI study. Gastroenterology. 2000;118:A615.
44. Tölle TR, Kaufmann T, Siessmeier T et al. Region-specific encoding of sensory and affective components of pain in the human brain: a positron emission tomography correlation analysis. Ann Neurol. 1999;45:40–7.
45. Frith C, Dolan R. The role of the prefrontal cortex in higher cognitive functions. Brain Res Cogn Brain Res. 1996;5:175–81.
46. Halsband U, Weyers M, Schmitt J, Binkofski F, Grützner G, Freund HJ. Recognition and imitation of pantomimed motor acts after unilateral parietal and premotor lesions: a perspective on apraxia. Neuropsychologia. 2000 (In press).
47. Wietek B, Lotze M, Hinninghofen H, Jehle EC, Grodd W, Enck P. Cortical activation during anorectal stimulation in patients with ulcerative colitis prior and after proctocolectomy. Digestion. 2001;63:278.
48. Kern MK, Arndoerfer RC, Shaker R. Cerebral cortical registration of rectal distension below perception threshold. Gastroenterology. 2000;118:A445.
49. Nour S, Svarer C, Kristensen JKI, Paulson OB, Law I. Cerebral activation during micturition in normal men. Brain. 2000;123:781–9.
50. Hamdy S, Aziz Q, Rothwell JC et al. Explaining oropharyngeal dysphagia after unilateral hemisperic stroke. Lancet. 1997;350:686–91.
51. Aziz Q, Phillips ML, Gregory LJ et al. Modulation of the brain processing of human oesophageal sensations by emotions: a functional magnetic resonance imaging study. Gastroenterology. 2000;118:A385.

52. Ringel Y, Drossman DA, Turkington TG *et al*. Anterior cingulate cortex (ACC) dysfunction in subjects with sexual/physical abuse. Gastroenterology. 2000;118:A80.
53. Ladabaum U, Minoshima S, Hasler WL, Cross D, Chey WD, Owyang C. Gastric distension correlates with activation of multiple cortical and subcortical regions. Gastroenterology. 2001;120:369–76.
54. Faas F, Feinle C, Enck P, Grundy D, Boesiger P. Central modulation of gastric motor activity. Am J Physiol. 2001;280:G850–7.
55. Liu Y, Gao JH, Liu GL, Fox PT. The temporal response of the brain after eating revealed by functional MRI. Nature. 2000;405:1058–62.
56. Fukudo S, Kano M, Hamaguchi T *et al*. Role of histaminergic neurons in gut-distension induced brain activation in human. Gastroenterology. 2000;118:A630.
57. Diksic M, Nakai A, Kumakura Y, Biovin M, Kersey KE. Regional brain serotonin synthesis in male and female irritable bowel syndrome (IBS) patients. Gastroenterology. 2000;118:A80.
58. Nabiloff BD, Chang L, Mandelkern M, Hamm L, Mayer EA. Evidence for selective effects of the 5HT3 antagonist alosetron on amygdala and hippocampal activation in IBS patients. Gastroenterology. 2000;118:A81.

2
Minilaparoscopy – a new diagnostic tool

J. M. ZEEH, U. TREICHEL and G. GERKEN

INTRODUCTION

Early in the 20th century laparoscopy was introduced[1] as a medical tool and, over years and decades, it has become an important diagnostic procedure for the internist (Table 1). In the 1970s various non-invasive techniques such as ultrasound, computerized tomography and, later, magnetic resonance imaging became standard procedures. Finally rapid technical improvements in these methods made them superior over diagnostic laparoscopy.

On the other hand, laparoscopic optics and accessories have always been subject to continuous technical improvement and miniaturization since more minimally invasive surgical procedures were performed.

With the introduction of minilaparoscopy in the 1990s this technique again attracted interest in the field of internal medicine, particularly for gastroenterologists[2–5]. Optics with a diameter less than 2 mm make minilaparoscopy a minimally invasive procedure which can be performed in analgosedation under ambulant conditions.

For the diagnosis and staging of liver diseases, and for the inspection of the peritoneum, minilaparoscopy appears to be the most rapid and sensitive interventional method[6,7]. In combination with a liver biopsy minilaparoscopy provides higher diagnostic safety than any other procedure. The possibility to effectively

Table 1 History of laparoscopy

1910	First laparoscopy in humans (Jacobaeus)
1930s	*Heinz Kalk* – Mentor of laparoscopy
1958	Menghini-technique of percutaneous biopsies
1970s	Introduction of medical ultrasound and computerized tomography
1980s	Introduction of magnetic resonance imaging
1996	Introduction of minilaparoscopy

control sustained bleeding after biopsy by monopolar coagulation of the tissue is another important advantage of this method. Therefore patients at high risk of bleeding can also undergo an invasive diagnostic work-up, which in the past has always been considered a contraindication.

The entire spectrum of minilaparoscopy comprises the inspection of abdominal organs, masses and the peritoneum (Table 2). Early stages of portal hypertension may be diagnosed by visualization of prominent smaller mesenteric vessels. Examination conditions are restricted if patients have adhesions of extensive mesenteric fat tissue. Due to the small size of the working trocars, and the fragility of the optic and instruments, there are only limited possibilities for adhesiolysis or mobilization of intra-abdominal fat.

INDICATIONS

Laparoscopy is the most reliable method for the diagnosis of liver diseases such as cirrhosis, and is superior to ultrasound or computerized tomography. Therefore it is also a valuable tool for initial staging, and to follow the course of a liver disease. Masses or lesions of the liver and spleen can be diagnosed, biopsied or further explored in most cases when no or little manipulation is necessary. Mild forms of portal hypertension may not be detected by abdominal ultrasound, duplex sonography or endoscopy. Minilaparoscopy, however, allows inspection of smaller portal vessels which might appear prominent. Lesions of the peritoneum can easily be seen and biopsied by minilaparoscopy. This is particularly important to rule out metastatic disease of the peritoneum, or for the diagnosis of tuberculosis. In cases of splenomegaly or fever of unknown origin minilaparoscopy may provide important information; in acute liver failure a preexisting liver disease can be discriminated from an acute episode, which is essential for the therapeutic approach.

For a synopsis of the indications see Table 3.

Table 2 Options of minilaparoscopy

Inspection and/or biopsy:
  Abdominal organs
  Abdominal masses
  Vessels
  Peritoneum
Controlled biopsies

Table 3 Indications for minilaparoscopy

Staging and grading of liver diseases
Masses or lesions of the liver or spleen
Portal hypertension
Lesions of the peritoneum
Obscure splenomegaly
Increased biopsy risk (bleeding)
Acute liver failure

PREPARATION AND EXAMINATION

Minilaparoscopy can be performed in a normal endoscopy environment. The patient should be fixed to an adjustable operation table and under ECG and pulsoxymetric monitoring. The examination is performed by two physicians (or a physician and an experienced nurse); one nurse is needed for non-sterile assistance. The examiners wear a face mask, cap, sterile coat and gloves after hand disinfection. The equipment will be set up on a table next to the assistant (shown in Figure 1a and 1b).

The patient must give written consent; actual blood tests are mandatory. If thrombocytes are <40/nl and/or TPZ<40% adequate substitution is recommended.

Prior to the examination liver and spleen should be located by abdominal ultrasound to avoid accidental puncture. The patient receives mild analgosedation with pethidin and midazolam in an initial dose of 50 mg and 1–2 mg, respectively.

After skin disinfection and local anaesthesia the peritoneum is punctured with a Verres needle (paraumbilical, 2 cm craniolateral left, Figure 2). The pneumoperitoneum is created by N_2O given through the Verres needle. Then the Verres needle is removed and the optic with the camera introduced through a remaining trocar (Figure 3). Inspection of all abdomial organs is now possible. If liver biopsy needs to be performed another incision is made in the right upper abdomen and the peritoneum is punctured with a second needle under laparoscopic control. Through a

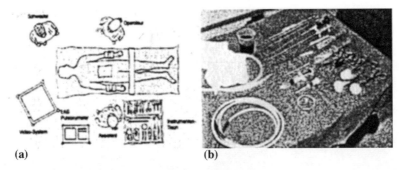

Figure 1 Minilaparotomy equipment

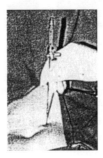

Figure 2 Puncture of the peritoneum with Verres needle

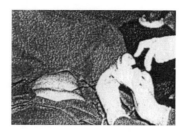

Figure 3 Introduction of optic and camera

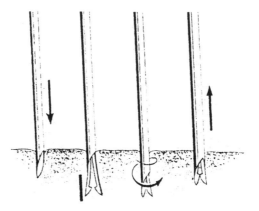

Figure 4 Liver biopsy with Silverman needle

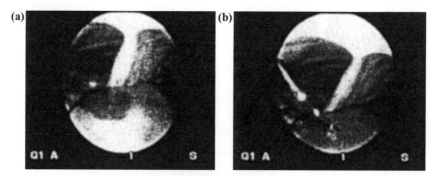

Figure 5 (a) Biopsy site; (b) monopolar coagulation

trocar biopsies can be taken with either a small forceps or a biopsy needle (e.g. Silverman needle, Figure 4). After biopsy the bleeding usually stops within 2 min. In case of persistent bleeding the biopsy site can be coagulated by a monopolar electrical probe (Figure 5). Minor manipulations can be done through the second trocar in the right upper quadrant to mobilize the liver lobes or fat tissue on the liver or spleen. To terminate the examination the trocars are removed after releasing the gas. Due to the small incisions no suturing is required.

After the procedure we keep the patient in bed for 4h under monitoring of pulse and blood pressure. Then the patient can be mobilized and can eat.

PATIENTS AND DIAGNOSES

In the past 2 years, in our Division of Gastroenterology and Hepatology at the University of Essen, 293 minilaparoscopic examinations have been performed and evaluated. The age of the patients was between 10 and 80 years. The majority (50%) was between 40 and 60 years old; 57% were male, 43% were female. The indications for minilaparoscopy in these patients are shown in Table 4: 59% had hepatitis (82% viral, 18% autoimmune); 15% had primary biliary cirrhosis and 7% had primary sclerosing cholangitis; 13% of the patients suffered from unknown liver disease.

The mean duration of the examination was 22 min. An additional 47 min were needed for general preparation, cleaning, sterilization, instrument set-up and patient care prior to and after the procedure.

The macroscopic diagnoses in these patients were cirrhosis in 50%, fibrosis in 25% and steatosis in 7%. A normal liver was seen in 10% of the patients. In 4% we saw masses like hepatocellular carcinoma, focal nodular hyperplasia, abscesses etc. (Table 5).

Pethidin and midazolam were given for analgesia and sedation prior to the examination. The required doses were quite different (Table 6). The majority of the patients received 3 mg midazolam and 50 mg pethidin.

The majority of our patients had normal blood tests; however, 28% had a thrombocyte count between 50 and 150/nl and 8% below 50/nl. The PTT was 40–70 s in 12% of patients and >70 s in 8%. The TPZ was 20–70% in 14% of patients and <20% in 3% of patients (Table 7).

Table 4 Indications (%)

Hepatitis	59
Hepatitis B	22
Hepatitis C	58
Hepatitis B+C	3
Autoimmune hepatitis	18
Primary biliary cirrhosis	15
Primary sclerosing cholangitis	7
Aliment/toxic	4
Wilson	2
Unknown liver disease	13

Table 5 Macroscopic diagnoses (%)

Cirrhosis	50
Fibrosis	25
Adhesions	4.5
Steatosis	7
Normal	14

Table 6 Analgosedation

Midazolam (mg)	Percentage	Pethidin (mg)	Percentage
0	19	0	1
1–3	27	25	2
4–5	46	50	93
7–8	7	75	1
>8	1	100	2

Table 7 Blood tests

Test	Percentage
Thrombocytes (per nanolitre)	
<50	8
50–150	28
150–450	61
>450	2
TPZ (%)	
<20	3
20–70	14
>70	83
PTT (s)	
>70	8
40–70	12
<40	80

Table 8 Macroscopic versus microscopic comparisons

Macroscopic	Microscopic
16 × Cirrhosis	16 × Cirrhosis
5 × Normal	5 × Normal
2 × Normal	Fibrosis
4 × Cirrhosis	Fibrosis
2 × Fibrosis	Normal
1 × Fibrosis	No diagnosis

MACROSCOPIC AND MICROSCOPIC DIAGNOSES

In a subset of 30 patients we compared the macroscopic diagnosis obtained by minilaparoscopy with the histological diagnosis (Table 8). In 16 cases both minilaparoscopy and histology described a complete cirrhosis and in five cases a normal liver. In four patients a cirrhosis was diagnosed macroscopically by minilaparoscopy whereas histology has only seen a fibrosis in the biopsies. In three cases where minilaparoscopy described a fibrosis the pathologist saw normal liver tissue in two cases and could not make a diagnosis in one case. In two patients minilaparoscopy described a normal liver. In these cases the histological examination revealed a fibrosis.

These results clearly demonstrate that the macroscopic evaluation of the organ by minilaparoscopy is more sensitive in detecting liver disease. These findings are supported by earlier studies[8–10] which found that only in 58–77% of the histological results did the liver biopsy correspond with the macroscopic diagnosis. There is a mismatch between the diagnosis, especially in early Child A stages and in macronodular cirrhosis[9,16].

COMPLICATIONS

Complications during minilaparoscopy occurred in 3% of cases. None of the patients who developed complications died during or after the examination. Vagal reactions with bradycardia and a drop in blood pressure were seen in five patients. In all cases an injection of atropine could control the symptoms, and this allowed us to continue the examination. One patient with a history of coronary heart disease started to suffer from angina pectoris after puncture of the peritoneum. Although intravenous application of nitroglycerine caused quick relief, we decided to stop the examination in this case. One young patient with an unknown liver disease and no other medical history developed cardiac arrest. He could be successfully resuscitated after 15 s. In this case we also stopped the examination. In one patient we accidentally punctured the stomach; in a second one the colon. In both cases patients received intravenous antibiotics. None of them developed fever or peritonitis, and both could be dismissed the next day.

Previous studies have reported complications during laparoscopy in 0.7–7.4% of cases[8,11,12]. Therefore the complication rate of 3% which we observed seems to be a realistic number. Mortality in our patients was zero. Other studies reported a mortality rate between 0% and 0.5%[11,13].

SUMMARY AND PERSPECTIVES

Minilaparoscopy is a new tool in the hands of gastroenterologists and a renaissance of conventional laparoscopy[2,4,5]. Instrument sizes being less than 2 mm in diameter allows a safe and quick inspection of all abdominal organs and of tumours. Minilaparoscopic-guided liver biopsies are of better quality compared to percutaneous biopsies, which leads to a lower number of false-negative histological results[14]. In combination with a liver biopsy minilaparoscopy provides high diagnostic safety for liver diseases and represents the gold standard for the diagnosis of liver cirrhosis[8,15]. Although histology confirms the macroscopic diagnosis in most cases, histology alone tends to underestimate the grade of liver fibrosis and cirrhosis[8–10].

Patients at high risk for bleeding can undergo this procedure due to its minor invasiveness. In case of continuous bleeding after liver biopsy this method allows easy control of the situation by coagulation of the biopsy site[3]. Furthermore, minilaparoscopy is an important tool in the clinical work-up of patients with intra-abdominal malignancies, including the diagnosis of peritoneal metastases. Further prospective studies need to be conducted to define new diagnostic and therapeutic options of this method. In combination with other techniques such as miniprobe endosonography, or by using flexible instruments, the diagnostic sensitivity and specificity of minilaparoscopy can be further improved in the hands of experienced interventional hepatogastroenterologists.

References

1. Kalk H. Erfahrungen mit der Laparoskopie. Z Klin Med. 1929:111–303.
2. Helmreich-Becker I, Gödderz W, Mayet WJ, Meyer zum Büschefelde KH, Lohse AW. Die Minilaparoskopie in der Diagnostik chronischer Lebererkrankungen. Endoskopie heute. 1997; 2:195–7.
3. Helmreich-Becker I, Meyer zum Büschefelde KH, Lohse AW. Safety and feasibility of a new minimally invasive diagnostic laparoscopy technique. Endoscopy. 1998;30:756–62.
4. Nader AK, Jeffers LJ, Reddy RK et al. Small-diameter (2 mm) laparoscopy in the evaluation of liver disease. Gastrointest Endosc. 1998;48:620–3.
5. Mössner J. Laparoscopy in der internistischen Differentialdiagnostik. Z Gastroenterol. 2001(Suppl. 39):1–6.
6. Gaiani S, Gramantieri L, Venturoli N et al. What is the criterion for differentiating chronic hepatitis from compensated cirrhosis? A prospective study comparing ultrasound and percutaneous liver biopsy. J Hepatol. 1997;27:979–85.
7. Cardi M, Muttillo IA, Amadori L et al. Superiority of laparoscopy compared to ultrasonography in diagnosis of widespread liver diseases. Dig Dis Sci. 1997;42:546–8.
8. Vido I, Wildhirt E. Korrelation des laparoskopischen und histologischen Befundes bei chronischer Hepatitis und Leberzirrhose. Dtsche Med Wochenschr. 1969;94:1633–7.
9. Helmreich-Becker I. Minilaparoskopie in der Leberdiagnostik – ein Vorteil? Z. Gastroenterology. 2001(Suppl. 39):7–9.
10. Poniachik J, Bernstein DE, Reddy R et al. The role of laparoscopy in the diagnosis of cirrhosis. Gastrointest Endosc. 1996;43:568–71.
11. Orlando K, Lirussi F, Nassuato G, Okolicsanyi L. Complications of laparoscopy in the elderly: a report of 345 consecutive cases and comparison with a younger population. Endoscopy. 1987;19:145–6.
12. Adamek HE, Maier M, Benz C, Huber T, Schilling D, Riemann JF. Schwerwiegende Komplikationen der Laparoskpie. Med Klin. 1996;91:694–7.
13. Kane MG, Krejs GJ. Complications of diagnostic laparoscopy in Dallas: a 7 year prospective study. Gastrointest Endosc. 1984;30:237–40.
14. Nord HJ. Biopsy diagnosis of cirrhosis: blind percutaneous versus guided direct vision techniques. Gastrointest Endosc. 1982;28:102–4.
15. Pagliaro L, Rinaldi F, Craxi A et al. Percutaneous blind biopsy versus laparoscopy with guided biopsy in diagnosis of cirrhosis. A prospective randomized trial. Dig Dis Sci. 1983;28:102–4.
16. Kameda Y, Asakawa H, Shimomura S et al. Laparoscopic prediction of hepatocellular carcinoma in cirrhosis patients. J Gastroenterol Hepatol. 1997;12:921–5.

3
Laparoscopy and endoscopy – competitive or complementary?

H. FEUSSNER and E. FRIMBERGER

INTRODUCTION

Laparoscopy is one of the oldest forms of endoscopy. In use for long time for the exploration of internal organs, mainly the liver, it gradually lost importance with the arrival of modern imaging techniques such as ultrasonography (US) and computerized tomography (CT) or magnetic resonance imaging (MRI). Eighty years after the invention of this procedure it was rediscovered again not only as a diagnostic but also as a therapeutic tool. This renaissance of laparoscopy, however, was stimulated not by internists but by surgeons. Gastroenterologists now are mainly devoted to flexible (intraluminal) endoscopy and continuously extend the range of endoluminal interventions. This may stimulate some competition among gastroenterologists and surgeons: former surgical domains are more and more invaded by less traumatic endoluminal procedures. Conversely, surgeons have also to admit that minor-access surgery, in particular cholecystectomy, was possible only due to concomitant endoscopic support ('therapeutic splitting').

Despite the undeniable advantages of endoluminal endoscopy some specific drawbacks must still be accepted: some regions of the gastrointestinal tract such as the small bowel are not yet accessible for the endoscope. Endoscopic treatment is possible only in the case of superficial lesions. Haemostasis is still difficult and tissue approximation from within the lumen is not yet feasible. Therefore, conventional surgery is still indicated in the majority of cases. Nevertheless, efforts should be made to make treatment less invasive and less traumatic than it is today.

Minor-access surgery is less traumatic than open surgery and offers a direct approach to practically all internal organs. The precise localization, especially of early lesions, however, is sometimes difficult due to the loss of the third dimension.

Combining the laparoscopic approach with a simultaneous endoscopic examination could help to overcome the specific drawbacks of each method[1-3]. A considerable number of case reports and studies has demonstrated that the range of minimally invasive approaches can thus be widened[4-10].

We systematically evaluated, in our own series of 112 patients with various gastrointestinal lesions, the technical aspects and clinical impact of combined intracavitary/endoluminal interventions.

METHODS AND PROCEDURES

Videolaparoscopy was performed by a Storz OR 1 (Storz, Tuttlingen, Germany) system. A 10 mm 30° telescope was used. For endoluminal endoscopy last-generation flexible endoscopes (GIF Q 140 gastroscope, CF 140 colonoscope, Olympus, Hamburg, Germany) were required to avoid the endoscope being blinded by the laparoscope. Four different screens were required to visualize both the endoluminal and laparoscopic scenario for the endoscopist and the laparoscopist. In the last 20 cases the endoscopist used a new head-mounted display (EyeTrek, Olympus, Hamburg, Germany) which significantly facilitated a more ergonomic

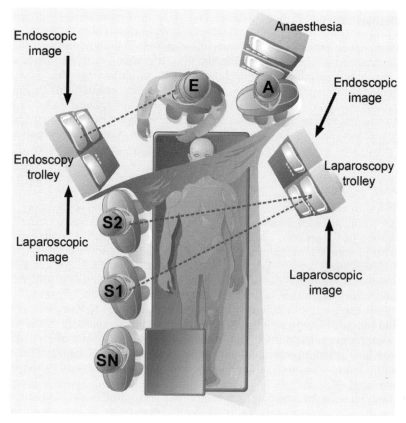

Figure 1 Positioning of the team and the equipment for combined laparoscopic/endoscopic procedures on the upper gastrointestinal tract. E, endoscopist; S, surgeon; SN, scrub nurse; A, anaesthesist

LAPAROSCOPY AND ENDOSCOPY – DO THEY TRAVERSE?

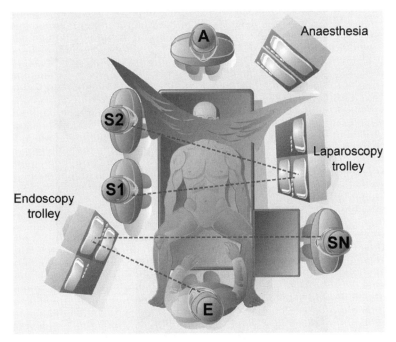

Figure 2 Positioning of the team and the required hardware for combined interventions on the colon. For the endoscopist the (additional) use of a head-mounted display has turned out to be helpful. E, endoscopist; S, surgeon; SN, scrub nurse

position during the intervention and made one screen superfluous. The positioning of the team depended upon the target. In upper gastrointestinal lesions the endoscopist was placed at the head of the patient and the laparoscopic surgeon stood at the right side of the patient (Figure 1). For colonic procedures the patient was in a lithotomy position with the endoscopist sitting between the legs. The surgeon stood at the opposite side of the lesion (Figure 2).

The combined approach was performed either as a laparoscopically assisted endoscopic procedure or as an endoscopically assisted procedure. Accordingly, four different approaches are possible.

1. Laparoscopically assisted endoscopic resection (LAER): LAER was chosen if endoscopic resection seemed to be possible in principle, but if the risk of perforation or bleeding, or incomplete resection, was considered too high. By simultaneous laparoscopy the lesion was brought into an optimal position for endoscopic resection, and endoluminally removed with a snare. In the case of an imminent perforation the site of resection could easily be oversewn or closed with a stapling device (Figure 3).

2. Endoscopically assisted wedge resection (EAWR): a wedge resection could be performed if the lesion was localized at the anterior gastric wall and the greater curvature or the antimesocolic side of the colon. The lesion was elevated with two stay sutures under endoscopic control, and removed using the linear stapling device (Figure 4).

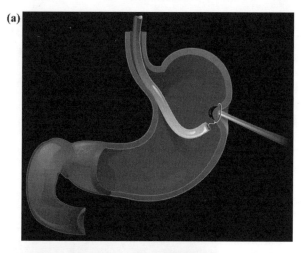

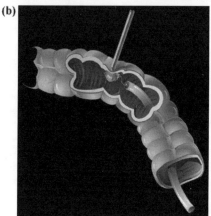

Figure 3 The principles of the laparoscopically assisted endoscopic resection (LAER): (a) stomach, (b) colon. Under endoscopic guidance the tumour site is protruded into the lumen with a laparoscopic pushing rod. Thus, a very good exposure of the lesion and of its surroundings is achieved, which facilitates application of the snare, and allows complete excision of the lesion, including safety margins. In case of perforation or imminent perforation the site can easily be oversewn laparoscopically

3. Endoscopically assisted transluminal resection (EATR): if the lesion was found at the posterior wall of the stomach, or at the mesocolic side of the colon, the lumen had to be opened by a small incision corresponding to the exact position of the lesion. Endoscopic guidance was essential for this manoeuvre. The lesion was elevated, removed with the stapling device and, finally, the incision was closed again (Figure 5).
4. Endoscopically assisted segmental resection (EASR): segmental resection of the (distal) stomach or the colon was necessary in circumferential or very large lesions which could not be managed by an alternative method.

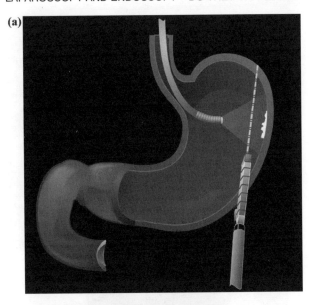

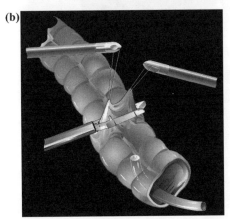

Figure 4 Endoscopically assisted laparoscopic wedge resection (EAWR): (**a**) stomach, (**b**) colon. The position of the lesion must be identified and demonstrated by the endoscopist. Oralad and caudad stay sutures are applied by the laparoscopist. The respective area is now elevated and resected by means of a linear stapler

As shown, the role of endoscopy was not confined to an exact localization of the lesion. The decision of how to proceed (LAER, EAWR, EATR, or EASR) depends entirely upon the intraoperative endoscopic aspect. In LAER both the resection and specimen retrieval are performed endoscopically (Table 1). Furthermore, simultaneous endoscopy is invaluable to avoid stenoses, in particular if the lesion is found in the vicinity of the cardia or pylorus, or in the colon.

With slight modifications these procedures were applied in benign disease and early malignant conditions of the oesophagus, stomach, duodenum and small

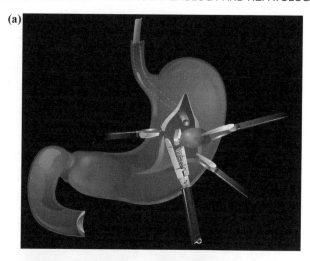

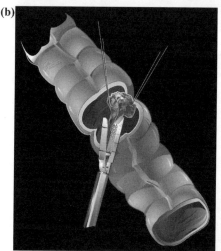

Figure 5 Endoscopically assisted transluminal resection (EATR): **(a)** stomach, **(b)** colon. A small enterotomy is performed close to the lesion which is supported by the endoscopist. The lesion is lifted up by forceps or stay sutures, and removed using a linear stapler. The enterotomy is then closed again. Reliable closure of the incision should be checked by the endoscopist (instillation of methylene blue)

Table 1 The role of endoscopy in combined endoscopic/laparoscopic procedures

1. Localization
2. Extent of resection
3. Decision-making concerning the appropriate surgical technique
4. Safety margins
5. Prevention of stenosis
6. Specimen retrieval

bowel, and the colon. If the tumour turned out to be more advanced than T1 mucosa (gastric cancer) or than T1 G2 (e.g. T3–4, infiltration of vessels, etc.) (colonic cancer), radical resection with lymphadenectomy was considered necessary.

OESOPHAGUS

The treatment of benign tumours of the oesophageal wall (GIST) or epiphrenic diverticula usually requires thoracotomy. Today a thoracoscopic procedure is feasible if the tumour is precisely located, which can easily be achieved using intraoperative oesophagoscopy. After removal the mucosa can be checked for integrity.

In epiphrenic diverticula, transhiatal laparoscopic resection is possible if supported by simultaneous endoscopy.

STOMACH

There is no doubt that endogastric lesions should preferably be treated by endoluminal endoscopy. In some cases, however, the lesion concerned is not suitable for endoscopic treatment alone. In these instances a laparoscopic approach could be helpful. By laparoscopy, local excision is possible. However, precise localization of the region of interest is essential, which can be provided only by simultaneous gastroscopy. Other than localization, gastroscopy is also helpful to avoid stenosis and to evaluate results of the laparoscopic procedure.

COLON

The treatment of colonic lesions is an important additional field for combined procedures. In the majority of cases of benign or premalignant lesions, colonoscopic polypectomy is the treatment of choice. In some cases, however, endoscopic removal can be too difficult or too dangerous (incomplete resection, bleeding, perforation). Instead of open surgical resection, combined colonoscopic/laparoscopic interventions could be an attractive alternative.

It is often argued that preoperative dye staining may be as helpful as intraoperative colonoscopy. Under practical conditions, however, staining is less reliable than expected. Furthermore, intraoperative endoscopy offers valuable additional support such as prevention of stenoses or examination of the wound closure.

OUR OWN RESULTS

Up to now, 112 combined procedures have been performed in 59 male and 53 female patients. Median age was 64 years (range 28–88). The majority of the lesions was located in the colon and stomach. Thirteen operations had to be performed on the oesophagus and three upon the duodenum and small bowel (Table 2). LAER was the leading procedure in four cases, EAWR in 44 cases, EATR in 44 and EASR in another 14 instances. In six patients the procedure had to be converted.

Table 2 Localization of the lesions, and leading procedures used

Localization of lesions	Leading procedure
Oesophagus ($n = 13$)	EAWR ($n = 13$)
Stomach ($n = 35$)	LAER ($n = 2$), EAWR ($n = 15$), EATR ($n = 18$)
Duodenum ($n = 2$)	LAER ($n = 1$), EAWR ($n = 1$)
Small bowel ($n = 1$)	EASR ($n = 1$)
Caecum ($n = 17$)*	EAWR ($n = 2$), EATR ($n = 9$), EASR ($n = 6$)
Ascending colon ($n = 13$)†	EAWR ($n = 6$), EATR ($n = 7$)
Transverse colon ($n = 11$)*	EAWR ($n = 4$), EATR ($n = 7$)
Descending colon ($n = 6$)*	EAWR ($n = 2$), EATR ($n = 1$), EASR ($n = 3$)
Rectosigmoid ($n = 13$)	LAER ($n = 1$), EAWR ($n = 1$), EATR ($n = 2$), EASR ($n = 4$)

* One conversion.
† Three conversions.

Perioperative complications occurred in nine patients (8%). Leakage of the anastomosis was seen in four patients, and reoperation was necessary in one. The patient who had to be reoperated had had to be converted to an open segmental resection. An ileostomy was done 7 days after the first operation. The patient died 3 days later because of general organ insufficiency. In two patients local inflammation of the trocar site was observed. One patient presented with severe cardiac ischaemia 6 days after laparoscopic wedge resection. Immediate dilation and stenting was performed and the patient survived. Another patient presented a leakage of the gastric stapler line and had to be reoperated; another one suffered a severe endoluminal gastric bleeding which could not be controlled endoscopically.

Reoperations for oncological reasons had to be done in six patients in whom definitive histopathological examination of the specimen revealed a more advanced tumour stage than originally assumed, although an intraoperative frozen-section examination had been performed. In two of these six patients a T2 carcinoma was found. Lymph node infection was present in one patient.

The hospital stay was 3 days for laparoscopically assisted endoscopic resection, 7 days for the wedge resection and 11 days for transluminal resection. To the present no regional recurrences have been observed.

CONCLUSIONS

Combined laparoscopic–endoscopic procedures are technically demanding and depend upon sophisticated hardware and well-trained staff. Coordination of the surgeon and gastroenterologists is not always easy. Intraoperative endoscopy, in particular colonoscopy, is far more difficult than under normal conditions, since some shortcomings (changing of the patient's position, bowel preparation) are inevitable. Nevertheless, endoscopy could be performed successfully in all cases. The need for additional hardware increases crowding in the operation room, and the staff must manage additional tasks.

Our results demonstrate, however, that combined endoluminal/endocavitary approaches are feasible, and at least as safe as an open procedure.

Although this series, covering 112 patients, is one of the largest groups published up to now, it is pointed out that the learning curve is not yet complete, due to the small number of patients in the subgroups. With increasing experience it is possible to assume that results can be continuously improved. It is too early yet to advance an argument concerning the real benefits for the patient or for the health system. We have merely compared, based on a matched-pair analysis, the effects of combined and open approaches. Personal experience as gained to date, however, convinces us that the minor-access approach is superior with regard to postoperative pain, overall recovery, and cosmesis. This justifies the somewhat higher expenses for combined procedures. At any rate, combined procedures allow one to introduce entirely new, less traumatic interventions in various diseases of the gastrointestinal tract, which again confirms that laparoscopy and endoscopy should be considered as complementary rather than competitive options.

References

1. Feussner H, Allescher H.-D., Harms J. Rationale und Selektion für Kombinationsvorgehen bei Colondysplasien und T1 Carcinomen. Chirurgie. 2000;71:1202–6.
2. Ohgami M, Kumai K, Otani Y. Curative laparoscopic surgery for early gastric cancer: five years experience. World J Surg. 1999;23:187.
3. Sakuramoto S, Mieno H, Hiki Y. Intragastric mucosal resection assisted by endoscopy and laparoscopy. Endosc Dig. 1996;8:525.
4. Beck DE, Krauf RE. Laparoscopic assisted full thickness endoscopic polypectomy. Dis Colon Rectum. 1993;36:693.
5. Hiki Y, Sakuramoto S, Katada N, Shimao H. Kombiniertes laparoskopisch-endoskopisches Vorgehen beim Magencarcinom. Chirurgie. 2000;71:1193–201.
6. Kim J, Chung M, Shim M, Kwun K. Laparoscopic wedge resection of the caecum, assisted by colonoscopy. Coloproctology. 1996;18:158.
7. Reissman P, Tech TA, Piccirillo M, Nogueras JJ, Wexner SD. Colonoscopic assisted laparoscopic colectomy. Surg Endosc. 1994;8:1352.
8. Shallman RW, Shaw TJ, Roach JM. Colonoscopically assisted intracorporeal laparoscopic wedge resection of a benign right colon lesion. Surg Laparosc Endosc. 1993;3:482.
9. Smedh K, Skullman S, Kald A, Anderberg B, Nyström P-O. Laparoscopic bowel mobilization combined with intraoperative colonoscopic polypectomy in patients with inaccessible polyp of the colon. Surg Endosc. 1997;11:643.
10. Zuro LM, Mc Culloch CS, Saclarides TJ. Laparoscopic colotomy, polypectomy. Innovative minimally invasive procedure. AORN J. 1992;56:1068.

Section II
Image and evidence

4
Chronic pancreatitis: an evident role for endoscopy

J. DEVIÈRE and J.-M. DUMONCEAU

INTRODUCTION

Endoscopic drainage procedures of the main pancreatic duct (MPD) are currently proposed for chronic pancreatitis (CP) with morphologically demonstrable abnormalities. CP-related complications such as pseudocysts, which are also good indications for endotherapy, are discussed elsewhere in this book.

Endoscopic drainage procedures are indicated for patients presenting pain associated with lesions of CP classified as types II to V at pancreatography according to Cremer's classification[1] and corresponding to the severe grade of the Cambridge classification[2]. In patients with mild pancreatitis, endotherapy is of unproven efficacy and carries a higher risk compared to that performed in patients with more severe lesions[3]. Moreover, inserting a stent in a normal MPD may precipitate the development of morphological lesions compatible with the diagnosis of CP[4]. Patient selection for endotherapy in CP is important, and differences in such selection criteria probably account for discrepancies in clinical results reported by European and American groups of authors.

The aim of endotherapy in painful CP is to decompress the MPD, as is performed with surgical drainage procedures over a period of many years. The rationale for MPD decompression is to reduce the parenchymal pancreatic pressure, which is abnormally high in CP. Parenchymal hyperpressure results from duct obstruction and reduced compliance of the diseased, fibrotic, pancreas. This increased parenchymal pressure impairs capillary blood flow, and leads to ischaemia.

Benefits expected from MPD decompression are threefold: (1) to relieve pain (pain relief and relapse are associated with pressure decrease and increase, as demonstrated in longitudinal studies[5]; (2) to slow down the evolution towards atrophy[6,7] by stopping the process of secondary CP superimposed on primitive CP in areas upstream from the MPD obstacle, and (3) to restore the outflow of pancreatic juice into the duodenum via the papilla, so improving fat digestion.

This chapter reviews the medium- and long-term results reported by several independent groups of authors after endoscopic MPD drainage for CP, and describes the techniques used.

CLINICAL RESULTS

Pain

The results obtained after endotherapy in CP patients with MPD obstacles consisting of stone(s) alone and MPD stricture(s) (alone or associated with stones) are reviewed separately.

In our experience the MPD obstacle in CP consists of stone(s), stricture(s), or the association of both in 42%, 8%, and 50% of cases (unpublished results). These figures may differ from those observed in other centres, due to different referral patterns. Although the modalities and results of endotherapy in these different subgroups of patients are different, most series reported to date include all these types of patients (as well as patients with pseudocysts treated by cystoenterostomy!). This stems from the relatively low prevalence of the disease but also, unfortunately, from the relatively common practice in some centres of treating MPD stones by insufficient fragmentation (related to the use of inadequate lithotripsy techniques) and hence almost no extraction, followed by stent insertion to bypass stone fragments. These fragments rapidly obstruct the stent!

Patients with MPD stones but no stricture (Figure 1)

We have shown in a study including 70 patients with MPD stones but no stricture that the use of extracorporeal shockwave lithotripsy (ESWL) was the factor most closely associated with stone clearance ($p < 0.005$)[8]. Although the presence of a single stone in the MPD ($p < 0.05$) and confinement of stones to the head of the pancreas ($p < 0.05$) were also associated with MPD clearance (as confirmed by other authors)[9], those latter associations were not found to be statistically significant when multivariate analysis was used. This reflects our clinical experience that, since ESWL has become available for pancreatic stones (in 1987 in our unit), number and location of stones are almost irrelevant to the success of MPD clearance. With ESWL, complete failure of stone clearance is very exceptional. As a result our selection criteria for endotherapy have become much larger with regard to stone number and location. A 'by-product' of the use of ESWL was an increase in the proportion of patients with partial stone clearance: stone fragments may be too numerous to be cleared completely, in contrast with a single stone being extracted intact without the use of ESWL. This has no clinical impact since, whether stone clearance is complete or partial, it was found to be highly associated with pain disappearance ($p < 0.01$). The observation that pain disappears after partial MPD clearance suggests that stone fragments remaining after endoscopic extraction generally do not obstruct the outflow of pancreatic juice into the duodenum, at least if these fragments are millimetre-size and no downstream stricture is present. This is further suggested by the finding by Ohara et al.[7] that ESWL alone for MPD stones (with no attempt at stone fragment removal) completely relieves pain in almost 80% of patients. In that study

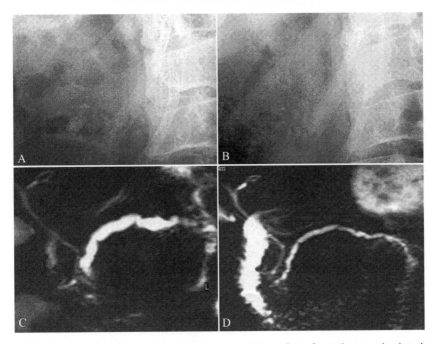

Figure 1 Decrease of MPD diameter and restoration of the outflow of exocrine secretion into the duodenum after (**D**), as compared to before (**C**) treatment. Before treatment (**A**) a single stone is detected in the area of the head of the pancreas at abdominal plain film; (**C**) the MPD is severely dilated, and no exocrine secretions appear in the duodenum after intravenous injection of secretin, as evidenced by magnetic resonance[16]. After treatment (**B**) few stone fragments are detected at abdominal plain film, (**D**) the MPD is much thinner, and exocrine secretions (in white) fill the duodenum shortly after intravenous injection of secretin

stone fragments spontaneously passed into the duodenum within 1 week in 75% of patients, as evidenced by serial abdomen X-ray and collection of stone fragments in stools.

With regard to long-term follow-up, the probability that our patients remained completely pain-free during 15 years after attempted stone extraction was 46%. Moreover, patients who did experience pain relapses nevertheless had the frequency of these pain attacks halved, in comparison to that observed before treatment. Interestingly, the patients who remained pain-free during the first 2 years following endotherapy very rarely experienced pain relapses. The proportion of patients who proceeded to surgery due to failed MPD drainage (and were thus excluded from the analysis of long-term results) was 5%.

Multivariate statistical analysis showed that three factors were independently associated with pain recurrence. These were: (1) the late performance of endotherapy during the course of the disease, (2) the presence of a MPD substenosis (i.e. judged too mild to require stenting), and (3) a high frequency of pain attacks before treatment. Noticeably, the persistence of stone fragments in the MPD at the end of endotherapy was not associated with pain relapse, further suggesting that small stone fragments may be eliminated spontaneously. Misunderstanding of that important fact is only one of the explanations for the inappropriate conclusions drawn by Adamek et al. in their study of 80 CP patients treated with ESWL and endoscopy[9]. These conclusions are in sharp contradiction with the data presented in that study (e.g. 'pancreatic drainage by endoscopy and ESWL has almost no effect on pain in chronic pancreatitis' although 61/80 (76%) patients reported 'complete or considerable pain relief' during a follow-up period of 40 months). Other explanations include a lack of precision (e.g. number of patients treated with pancreatic stents not stated), and inappropriate definition of successful treatment.

Patients with MPD strictures (associated or not with MPD stones)

Two approaches have been proposed for these patients, which yielded different results.

One of these approaches[10] consisted in inserting a 10-French (F) stent into the MPD stricture for a fixed duration (i.e. 6 months), after a rather aggressive stricture dilation procedure (i.e. inflating a 6-mm diameter balloon inside the stricture and repeating this procedure if a residual stricture was evidenced during stent exchange procedures performed 2, 4, and 6 months later). Intakes of analgesics could be discontinued immediately after stent insertion in 74% of the patients. However, this proportion dropped to 52% at 1 year after stent removal. At this time a persistent MPD stricture was evidenced at repeat pancreatography in 100% of patients taking analgesics, compared to 33% of those who did not ($p < 0.005$). Most importantly, this persistent MPD stricture was already visible immediately after stent removal in 82% of patients who would require analgesics 1 year later, compared to 25% of those who would not ($p < 0.05$). This study confirms the common clinical observation that the evolution of abdominal pain closely parallels that of MPD obstacles, and demonstrates that stenting should not be discontinued until a satisfactory stricture dilation is evidenced.

Rather than stenting MPD strictures for fixed duration, other authors[11–13,17] have proposed maintaining stenting until stricture dilation is obtained. Criteria of satisfactory stricture dilation have been defined. These are evaluated immediately after stent removal and include: (1) a rapid (less than 2 min) outflow of contrast medium into the duodenum after ductal filling upstream from the dilated stricture (note that results may vary according to the patient's position or after secretin injection); (2) easy passage of a slightly inflated extraction balloon catheter through the dilated stricture; and (3) disappearance of MPD dilation upstream from the dilated stricture (this latter criterion has been proposed by the group of Huibregtse et al. only, and we think that it does not reflect a satisfactory stricture dilation, but rather the fact of whether the stent was functional or not at the time of removal).

Using these criteria to decide when to interrupt stenting, satisfactory long-term results were reported in two studies including a total of 144 patients[12,13]: 87% and 100% of patients who had experienced pain relief immediately after stent insertion had sustained improvement during mean follow-up periods of 3.8 and 4.9 years after the first stent insertion. Seventy-two per cent of the patients discontinued the intake of analgesic and 75% had a weight gain greater than 5%[13]. In both studies the pain relief immediately after stent insertion was more frequent if endotherapy was applied earlier during the course of the disease, although the difference was not statistically significant. Criteria of satisfactory stricture dilation were fulfilled and stents were removed in two-thirds of cases, after mean stenting duration of 6[12] and 16[13] months. Stenting durations were 3 times longer in patients who did not fulfil these criteria[12]. This suggests that about one-third of MPD strictures are not amenable to dilation. Strictures relapsed after stent removal and required repeat stenting in 20% of cases. The results reported by Laugier et al.[14] in a small group of patients treated with either 7-F or 12-F stents suggest that 7-F stents are not effective in dilating MPD strictures.

Of the patients with MPD strictures 22–26% were excluded from the analysis of long-term results in these studies, due to continued pain. These percentages are relatively high compared to that reported in patients with MPD stones but no strictures (i.e. 5%)[8]. This difference probably relates: (1) to technical factors: the success rate of stone fragmentation is higher than that of stent insertion (99 vs. 85%)[10,15] (stone fragmentation provides at least partial MPD drainage)[7]; and (2) to the severity and duration of the disease, which is more important in patients with stones and strictures compared to those with stones alone.

STENT-RELATED COMPLICATIONS

Mild to moderate[16] complications were reported in 55% of patients[12,13]. These complications were treated by uneventful stent exchange procedures, usually performed on an ambulatory basis. Severe complications were reported by Binmoeller et al. only, in 6% of their patients[13]. These complications consisted of pancreatitis and abscess formation related to stent. The authors themselves ascribed the occurrence of severe complications to their stent exchange policy (i.e. waiting for symptoms of stent dysfunction before proceeding to stent exchange). As stents can easily be exchanged on an ambulatory basis, we propose to proceed with stent exchange at regular intervals adapted on an individual basis (i.e. every 6–12 months), except for reliable patients who may be asked to arrange the stent exchange procedure by phone as soon as they experience symptoms of stent dysfunction.

Worsening of MPD abnormalities during the stenting period was reported by Ponchon et al.[10] in 13% of cases, but not by Smits et al.[12] or by Binmoeller et al.[13]. However, Ponchon et al. did not state whether the new MPD lesions were located in the portion of the duct that was in contact with the stent. We often observed the development of MPD strictures unrelated to stents, either in areas not in contact with the stent, or in patients devoid of endoscopic treatment. These lesions simply reflect the progression of the fibrotic process characteristic of CP. Another hypothesis is that the new lesions detected by Ponchon et al. were related to the rather aggressive technique of stricture dilation used by these authors (i.e. up to a diameter of 6 mm). The shape and length of stents used is also crucial, since the impaction of the proximal stent end into the pancreatic parenchyma may induce a local inflammatory process. It is therefore recommended that a range of different stents be readily available when performing endotherapy in CP patients, to fit every variation in anatomy.

Few data concerning the optimal duration of MPD stenting are available. Among the patients that we have followed for 5 years or more we have observed that persistent stricture dilation after stent removal is unusual. On the contrary, the morphology of the MPD often evolves to a type III according to Cremer's classification. Many of these patients remain pain-free without further MPD stenting. The absence of pain recurrence could be related to the so-called 'burn-out' of the pancreas, although neither diabetes nor steatorrhoea develops in some of these patients (this could be related to the early performance of the endoscopic treatment during the course of the disease: long-term results after endoscopic treatment are difficult to compare with those reported after surgical MPD drainage procedures). So, the idea that stenting (and associated stent exchange requirements) could be necessary for the whole lifetime might be revisited in the near future.

CONCLUSION

The indications of endoscopic treatment for painful CP are strictly limited to the severe types of pancreatitis where a ductal obstruction is demonstrated. This method has gained success over recent years and with minimal complications allows one to avoid or postpone surgery. Endotherapy has the major advantage of being possibly repeated without an increase in morbidity. This should be proposed relatively early in the course of the disease, i.e. as soon as an obstacle is evidenced on the MPD in order to decrease the rate of painful recurrences and to preserve exocrine function. It must be considered as an iterative treatment that can be adapted to successive problems occurring along the course of a chronic disease.

References

1. Cremer M, Toussaint J, Hermanus A et al. Les pancréatites primitives: classification sur base de la pancréatographie endoscopique. Acta Gastroenterol Belg. 1976;39:522–46.
2. Axon ATR, Classen M, Cotton P et al. Pancreatography in chronic pancreatitis: international definition. Gut. 1984;25:1107–12.
3. Lehman G, Sherman S. Pancreas divisum: diagnosis, clinical significance and management alternatives. Gastrointest Endosc Clin N Am. 1995;5:145–70.
4. Smith MT, Sherman S, Ikenberry S et al. Alterations in pancreatic ductal morphology following polyethylene pancreatic stent therapy. Gastrointest Endosc. 1996;44:268–75.
5. Ebbehoj N, Borly L, Bulow J et al. Evaluation of pancreatic tissue fluid pressure and pain in chronic pancreatitis. A longitudinal study. Scand J Gastroenterol. 1990;25:462–6.
6. Nealon WH, Towsend CM, Thompson JC. Operative drainage of the pancretic duct delays functional impairment in patients with chronic pancreatitis. Ann Surg. 1988;208:321–9.
7. Ohara H, Hoshino M, Hayakawa T et al. Single application extracorporeal shock wave lithotripsy is the first choice for patients with pancreatic duct stones. Am J Gastroenterol. 1996;91:1388–94.
8. Dumonceau JM, Devière J, Le Moine O et al. Endoscopic drainage in chronic pancreatitis associated with ductal stones: long-term results. Gastrointest Endosc. 1996;43:547–55.
9. Adamek HE, Jakobs R, Buttmann A et al. Long term follow up of patients with chronic pancreatitis and pancreatic stones treated with extracorporeal shock wave lithotripsy. Gut. 1999;45:402–5.
10. Ponchon T, Bory RH, Hedelius F et al. Endoscopic stenting for pain relief in chronic pancreatitis: results of a standardized protocol. Gastrointest Endosc. 1995;42:452–6.

11. Cremer M, Devière J, Delhaye M et al. Stenting in severe chronic pancreatitis: results of medium term follow-up in seventy-six patients. Endoscopy. 1991;23:171–6.
12. Smits ME, Badiga SM, Rauws EAJ et al. Long-term results of pancreatic stents in chronic pancreatitis. Gastrointest Endosc. 1995;42:461–7.
13. Binmoeller KF, Jue P, Seifert H et al. Endoscopic pancreatic stent drainage in chronic pancreatitis and a dominant stricture: long-term results. Endoscopy. 1995;27:638–44.
14. Laugier R, Renou C. Endoscopic ductal drainage may avoid resective surgery in painful chronic pancreatitis without large ductal dilatation. Int J Pancreatol. 1998;23:145–52.
15. Delhaye M, Vandermeeren A, Baize M et al. Extracorporeal shock wave lithotripsy of pancreatic calculi. Gastroenterology. 1992;102:610–20.
16. Cotton PB. Outcomes of endoscopy procedures: struggling towards definitions. Gastrointest Endosc. 1994;40:514–18.
17. Costamagna G, Gabbrielli A, Mutignani M et al. Extracorporeal shock wave lithotripsy of pancreatic stones in chronic pancreatitis: immediate and medium-term results. Gastrointest Endosc. 1997;46:231–6.

5
Endosonography – what are the diagnostic advantages?

R. H. HAWES

INTRODUCTION

There has been a tremendous evolution in endoscopic ultrasound (EUS) since its introduction in the early 1980s. New equipment has been introduced, the technique of EUS-guided fine needle aspiration (FNA) has been developed and there has been a refinement in the application of EUS for pancreatobiliary diseases. During the same period, competing imaging modalities such as computerized tomography (CT) scan and magnetic resonance imaging (MRI) have improved. The evolution of these technologies has impacted the application of EUS, and the purpose of this chapter is to provide an update on the present advantages of EUS and to explore how these advantages can be exploited by clinicians to improve their evaluation of patients with pancreaticobiliary diseases.

UNIQUE PROPERTIES OF EUS

The principal advantage of EUS is its superior resolution. Using the endoscope as the endosonographer's 'arm', the transducer can be positioned directly adjacent to the pancreas and the extrahepatic biliary tree, permitting the use of high-frequency ultrasound transducers. These transducers provide higher resolution imaging than can be achieved with CT or MRI. There is no question that the development of multi-headed CT scanners provides consistently better images than conventional machines. The multi-headed systems allow complete pancreatobiliary imaging in a single breath-hold (less motion artifact) while obtaining thin, overlapping cuts. Additionally, the speed and predictability of imaging allows improved coordination between contrast injection and imaging. All these factors result in better, more consistent CT images, but there remains a theoretical limit to image resolution that has not changed with the advent of these new machines. The same holds true for MRI, though the theoretical limits on resolution for MRI are actually better than CT. Whether new-generation MRI machines can approach these limits while remaining cost-effective in a clinical environment is as yet unknown. In summary, EUS has a fundamental advantage in that, for those parts of the pancreatobiliary tree that can be visualized, image resolution is unmatched by any radiological or magnetic resonance device.

The second advantage of EUS lies in the evolution of EUS FNA. EUS is moving closer and closer to complete integration between imaging and tissue acquisition. When imaging alone falls short, EUS-guided FNA can be performed immediately. The cytological and now molecular information that can be added to the imaging data is making EUS a very powerful diagnostic tool. With CT the initial examination is usually confined to imaging alone. Once the images are processed, if a decision is made to perform guided FNA, a repeat examination is required. The limits in resolution also come into play in that lesions not seen by CT obviously cannot be targeted for needle aspiration. MRI-guided biopsy has proven very difficult and is not relavent to all but a few academic centres around the world.

While the global advantage of EUS lies in its superior resolution and tissue-acquisition capability, the following is a systematic discussion of the role of EUS as it relates to particular pancreatobiliary diseases.

BILE DUCT STONES

EUS has been found to be a very sensitive test for the detection of bile duct stones. This was first reported by Edmundowicz et al.[1] but their report was quickly followed by a much larger French study[2]. In the French study endoscopic retrograde cholangiopancreatography (ERCP) and surgical exploration were used as gold standards and the sensitivity and negative predictive value for EUS in the detection of bile duct stones was found to be 97%. Both figures were significantly better than extracorporeal ultrasound and CT, which were also evaluated in the French study. Since these two initial reports there have been many subsequent ones expanding the experience with endosonography in the detection of bile duct stones[3-5]. For the most part these latter reports have confirmed the results from the earlier experience. It now appears clear that in experienced hands, using ERCP or intraoperative cholangiography as a gold standard, that EUS is quite accurate; probably equal to or better than either of the two tests to which it has been compared. Several important advantages for EUS have emerged from these studies. First, it appears that stone size has little effect on the ability of EUS to detect stones – this again is rationalized by the superior resolution of this technology. Second, small stones in a dilated duct can pose formidable problems for direct cholangiography. Poor mixing of contrast and bile, combined with the large volumes of contrast needed to fill the biliary tree, can obscure small stones. Neither of these factors affects EUS, providing an advantage for this technique when these circumstances are present. The advent of ultrasound probes that can be advanced over a guidewire may provide the best solution. Use of these catheters allows accurate detection of bile duct stones in patients with dilated ducts and/or small stones without requiring the patient to undergo two procedures. The additional advantage for US catheters is that they can effectively image the intrahepatic biliary tree – an area not seen by conventional EUS.

CHOLANGIOCARCINOMA

A number of reports have described the utility of EUS to stage cholangiocarcinoma. One study reported by Yasuda et al.[6] looked at EUS versus ERCP, ultrasound, CT and angiography in the visualization of common bile duct tumours. EUS and ERCP saw tumours in 10 of 10 patients while US, CT and angiography had a sensitivity of 50%, 40% and 50%, respectively. Proximal bile duct tumours involving the hilum and intrahepatic biliary tree are often poorly or incompletely visualized. The accuracy of EUS in staging biliary malignancy is modest. T-stage accuracy for common bile duct and common hepatic duct tumours is approximately 85% while the N-staging ranges from 55 to 75% in studies by Tio et al. and Mukai et al.[7,8]. Mitake and co-workers[9] looked at EUS in staging gallbladder carcinoma and found T-stage accuracy of 77% and an N-stage accuracy of 90%.

There is not a vast literature on using EUS for malignant biliary tract disease. In part this is because it is relatively rare, and patients with proximal bile duct tumours are generally not effectively imaged with EUS.

The introduction of intraductal ultrasound probes has provided a more effective tool to image and stage bile duct tumours. These are now available from a number of companies. Ultrasound frequencies incorporated into these catheters range from 12 to 30 MHz. Several catheters are designed to pass over a guidewire, thus obviating the need for sphincterotomy. There are several advantages of these probes over the standard radial scanning EUS instruments:

1. By virtue of the position within the bile duct, the probe naturally orients perpendicular to a process arising from the wall of the bile duct; this provides superior images.
2. The entire biliary tree can be examined.
3. Imaging and therapy (stenting, etc.) can be performed in one procedure.
4. Over-the-wire probes can be applied without requiring sphincterotomy, and therapeutic procedures such as stenting can proceed without losing cannulation.

A promising application is staging biliary cancers[10–12]. These catheters are especially useful in detecting hepatic artery and portal vein invasion. The accuracy of detecting vascular invasion with intraductal ultrasonography (IDUS) is over 90%[10]. When combined with cholangioscopy it approaches 100%.

PANCREATIC CANCER

CT scan must be considered the primary imaging modality in patients with suspected pancreatic tumours. This is the case because it is well standardized and widely available. The main question with regard to EUS is whether EUS adds anything to CT in the evaluation of these patients. In the past numerous studies have compared EUS to conventional CT in detecting and staging pancreatic cancer[13,14]. These studies have documented a superiority for EUS which is especially apparent for tumours <3 cm in diameter[15,16].

Another way to look at EUS is to look at its accuracy in predicting complete resection. Tio and Tytgat demonstrated that EUS has an accuracy of 67%, 91% and 71% for predicting if an operation would be curative, palliative or the cancer is not resectable at all[17]. Rosch et al. compared EUS to CT, ultrasound and angiography, and found the prediction of resectability to be 80%, 36%, 24% and 52%, respectively[18].

The advent of spiral CT, however, has improved CT detection and staging of pancreatic cancer and necessitated new comparisons between EUS and CT. Two papers have recently been published which address this issue[19,20]. In the Legmann et al. report, 30 patients with suspected pancreatic tumours underwent dual-phase spiral CT and EUS. The results for the detection and staging of pancreatic tumours are shown in Tables 1 and 2. Table 3 breaks down the results according to tumour size. In these examples there begins to be a separation between CT and EUS. These data serve to highlight the differences in resolution – lesion size has no effect on sensitivity or accuracy of EUS. Another study[20] found similar results.

Table 1 Spiral CT compared to EUS in the detection of pancreatic tumours[19]

	CT (%)	EUS (%)
Sensitivity	92	100
Specificity	100 (3/3)	33 (1/3)
PPV = positive predictive value	100	93
NPV = negative predictive value	60	100
Accuracy	93	93

Table 2 Spiral CT compared to EUS in staging pancreatic cancer[19] (percentages)

	CT		EUS	
	T = tumour	N = lymph node	T	N
Accuracy	86	77	90	86
Understage	10	14	5	10
Overstage	5	10	5	5

Table 3 CT compared to EUS in the detection and staging of pancreatic tumours according to tumour size[19]

	0–15 mm	15–35 mm	>35 mm
Detection			
CT	67	100	100
EUS	100	100	100
Staging			
CT	66	83	100
EUS	100	92	86

MEDICAL IMAGING IN GASTROENTEROLOGY AND HEPATOLOGY

Table 4 Proposed algorithm for diagnosing and staging pancreatic mass

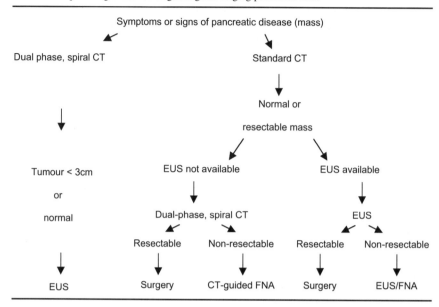

It must be pointed out that, while these studies demonstrate that differences in detection and staging accuracy for pancreatic tumours have narrowed between CT and EUS, most CT scans obtained 'in the community' are not performed with the rigorous techniques applied in these studies. The main advantages and disadvantages of each technique when applied to pancreatic tumours is summarized below:

1. EUS has the advantage for tumours ≤2 cm.
2. CT has the advantage for assessment of arterial invasion (arteries are tortuous and difficult to completely trace with EUS).
3. EUS has greater sensitivity in defining the relationship between the tumour and the portal vein for tumours <4 cm.
4. CT has the advantage in local staging of tumours >4 cm.
5. EUS has a significant advantage in lymph node (LN) detection.
6. CT has the advantage in detecting liver metastasis.

Given these principles, an algorithm is proposed for the application of EUS and CT in evaluating patients with suspected pancreatic tumours (Table 4).

CHRONIC PANCREATITIS

Making a diagnosis of advanced chronic pancreatitis is not difficult. However, patients with mild or moderate disease often have a normal CT and extracorporeal ultrasound. Some consider pancreatic function testing to be the gold standard, but it is difficult to perform and standardize, and few centres perform it well. Pancreatography with complete filling of secondary branches can diagnose early disease but this test is invasive, expensive and carries a real risk of pancreatitis. EUS sees the entire pancreas in the great majority of cases and has sufficient resolution to detect subtle abnormalities. The difficulty lies in the fact that there really is no true gold standard for the diagnosis of chronic pancreatitis. As a result, as clinicians have explored the use of EUS to detect early chronic pancreatitis, there has been no set standard with which to compare EUS, making the reliability of the results 'suspect'. It is the opinion of this author that the detection of early chronic pancreatitis provides one of the most significant 'niches' for EUS in the evaluation of pancreatic diseases, and the data to date will be systematically presented so that readers can form their own opinion.

In order to apply EUS to diagnose chronic pancreatitis, it is necessary to thoroughly understand the appearance of a 'normal' pancreas. Several studies have evaluated the pancreas in 'control' populations[21,22]. Nattermann et al.[21] reported EUS findings in 20 patients without suspected pancreatic disease and described the pancreatic parenchyma as 'homogeneous fine granular pattern with smooth margins'. Catalano et al.[22] reported on 25 'normal' patients and described the parenchyma as 'homogeneous and finely reticulated without evidence of side-branch ectasia'. A ventral anlage (echogenic difference between the ventral and dorsal pancreas) was seen in 68% of controls. No cysts or stones were described. The main pancreatic duct was uniformly tubular in shape with anechoic walls. Wiersema et al. evaluated the endosonographic features of a small group of healthy volunteers, with no prior history of abdominal pain or alcohol abuse[23]. The pancreatic parenchyma was 'uniform' and more echogenic than liver. A ventral anlage was detected in 45%. No cysts were seen. These data from control populations and healthy volunteers provide important standards for the normal endosonographic appearance of the pancreas, but the data may be considered limited due to the small numbers of patients and potential biases in the control populations.

Bill Lees is credited with describing the EUS features of chronic pancreatitis[24]. The characteristic findings (or criteria) include ductal and parenchymal changes, and are listed in Table 5.

A fundamental requirement for any test is reliability. When a gold standard does not exist, this is often measured as the degree to which practitioners agree on a diagnosis. Wiersema et al. compared the degree of agreement among three experienced endosonographers reading individual features of chronic pancreatitis[23]. Agreement ranged from 83 to 94% for various ductal and parenchymal features. To further improve the reliability an International Working Group has published

Table 5 Ultrasound features of chronic pancreatitis (adapted from ref. 24)

Ductal	Parenchymal
Echogenic walls	Echogenic foci
Irregular duct wall contour	Small cysts
Intraductal echogenic foci	Lobular outer contour
Side branch dilation	Echogenic strands
	Inhomogenicity

a set of Minimum Standard Terminology (MST) including definitions, for many of the EUS features of chronic pancreatitis[25]. Wallace et al. evaluated the interobserver reliability of EUS for the diagnosis of chronic pancreatitis by 11 highly experienced endosonographers. There was moderately good overall agreement for the final diagnosis of chronic pancreatitis ($\kappa = 0.45$) and for individual features of duct dilation ($\kappa = 0.6$) and lobularity ($\kappa = 0.51$) but poor for the other seven features ($\kappa < 0.4$). The expert panel had consensus or near-consensus agreement (>90%) on 206 of 450 (46%) individual exam features including 22 of 45 diagnoses of chronic pancreatitis[25]. Agreement in the EUS diagnosis of chronic pancreatitis is comparable to other commonly used endoscopic procedures such as bleeding ulcer stigmata ($\kappa = 0.34-0.66$)[26] and radiological procedures such as brain CT for stroke localization ($\kappa = 0.56-0.62$)[27] and better than the physical diagnosis of heart sounds ($\kappa = 0.05-0.18$)[28].

Few studies have compared EUS to histology in diagnosing chronic pancreatitis. Zimmerman et al. reported the EUS features in comparison to histological features of chronic pancreatitis in 34 patients who underwent EUS followed by pancreatectomy or open surgical biopsy (at the time of a lateral pancreaticoduodenostomy) (21 for chronic pancreatitis, 13 for pancreatic carcinoma)[29]. Overall 68% of patients met histological criteria for chronic pancreatitis. The total number of EUS features present was predictive of histological chronic pancreatitis. The sensitivity and specificity using a threshold diagnosis of ≥3 features were 87%, and 64%, for ≥4 features 78% and 73%, for ≥5 features 60% and 83%, for ≥6 features 43%, and 91%. From these results it was concluded that a threshold of ≥4 features was the optimal threshold.

ERCP is probably the test most widely applied to detect chronic pancreatitis so it makes sense to compare EUS with ERCP. Multiple studies have compared the results of EUS to ERP in patients with abdominal pain and suspected chronic pancreatitis[21–23,30,31]. Three of these studies used standardized EUS and ERP (Cambridge classification) grading systems and can be compared directly[21,22,31]. Each of these studies evaluated the pancreas for the presence of 9–11 described features, and then considered EUS to be abnormal if the total number of features exceeded a threshold number (e.g. ≥3, or ≥4, or ≥5). It is clear from these studies that EUS and ERP agree in approximately 80% of cases. In cases where they disagree, the vast majority (74%) are abnormal by EUS and normal by ERP. Only 26% of discrepancies were ERP abnormal but EUS normal. It is unknown if EUS is more sensitive to mild changes of chronic pancreatitis than ERP, or if EUS is 'overdiagnosing' early chronic pancreatitis. It has become clear, from all comparative studies to date, that there is an inverse relationship between sensitivity and specificity when reporting the EUS criteria for chronic pancreatitis. The smaller number of features required to 'diagnose' chronic pancreatitis, the better the sensitivity – but specificity suffers. Alternatively, if you set the threshold high (large number of criteria must be identified to diagnose chronic pancreatitis) specificity will be high, but sensitivity will suffer. There is great concern among the gastroenterology community against over-diagnosing chronic pancreatitis – due to fears that it will justify the use of narcotics to treat the pain. Additionally, many pancreatologists feel that two tests should agree (a structural and functional test) before making a diagnosis. These considerations have led us to begin reporting EUS for detecting chronic pancreatitis as a probability: 0–3 features = normal, 4 features = 'intermediate' probability of chronic pancreatitis, and ≥4 features = 'high' probability of chronic pancreatitis.

No large well-designed studies have compared EUS to pancreatic function tests in the diagnosis of chronic pancreatitis. The two best studies to date are in abstract form only, and have not been published after a peer-review process. The first one was presented at Digestive Disease Week (DDW) in 1998 and came from the Mayo Clinic[32]. It compared EUS to a function test that measures lipolytic activity from a duodenal aspirate. In their preliminary results, EUS appeared to over call chronic pancreatitis if the lipolytic activity was considered the accurate test. Zuccaro et al. from the Cleveland Clinic presented their results comparing EUS to the standard double-lumen secretin test[33]. They used the secretin test as the gold standard and divided patients into those with advanced and mild disease. They also compared the results for EUS depending on whether 4, 5 or 6 features were required to diagnose chronic pancreatitis. For those with mild disease, EUS had excellent specificity using any criteria (4, 5 or 6 features) but had only a 10% sensitivity when 4 features were seen and 0 sensitivity if 5 or 6 features were present. One of the problems with the Zuccarro et al. study is that the secretin test was used as the standard – therefore it is not really a comparative study. One can conclude from their data that function testing and EUS, by virtue of looking at different aspects of the pancreas (one is a functional test and the other is a structural test), are not appropriate to compare, or that the study is inconclusive because function testing is not a gold standard; especially for early chronic pancreatitis.

Natural history may be the most definitive gold standard for early chronic pancreatitis. A diagnosis of 'mild' chronic pancreatitis based on EUS, which then progresses to more severe chronic pancreatitis as diagnosed by other tests (EUS + ERP + functional test), is likely to be a correct diagnosis. Unfortunately, there are no data on the long-term natural history of 'mild' chronic pancreatitis diagnosed by EUS. Hastier et al. reported the short-term (mean 22 months) progression of pancreatic disease in 17 alcoholic patients with an abnormal EUS but a normal ERP[34]. Follow-up EUS examinations for 12–38 months did not identify any progression to more overt (ERP-positive) disease. It is likely, however, that patients who required more than 55 years (mean age of study patients was 55.5 years) to develop 'mild' disease, require more than 2–3 years to progress from mild to more severe disease. A cross-sectional study of alcoholic patients with and without abdominal pain, by Bhutani[35], showed that an EUS diagnosis of chronic pancreatitis (≥4 features) was positive in 89% of alcoholics with abdominal pain but also in 58% of alcoholics without pain, and 0% of control patients (non-alcoholic, no abdominal pain). Further long-term follow up data are needed.

The diagnosis of early (or mild) chronic pancreatitis can be quite difficult; it requires a degree of suspicion and then appropriate tests. Function testing can be done but is offered in only a few centres with expertise in pancreatic diseases. It is a difficult test for patients to tolerate and has not been thoroughly evaluated in patients with mild disease. ERCP is most widely available, but this exam is technically demanding, expensive and carries a very real risk of causing acute pancreatitis. EUS is a structural (as opposed to a functional) study which can image the parenchyma as well as the ductal system. Studies to date suggest that it can detect abnormalities in the pancreas not seen by any other imaging technique. Its application in diagnosing chronic pancreatitis deserves further study but, if available, it should be applied to patients with undiagnosed upper abdominal pain.

CONCLUSION

In conclusion, EUS has a particular niche in pancreatobiliary diseases, primarily because of its superior resolution. EUS sees small processes well. It appears to be an excellent modality to detect bile duct stones but the major question that remains is: in what clinical context should it be applied? Emerging indications may include gallstone pancreatitis and in some cases prelaparoscopic cholecystectomy when there is a moderate to low probability of bile duct stones – especially if intraoperative cholangiography is not possible. Catheter probes have emerged as being quite useful in the evaluation of patients with bile duct tumours and may be used as an adjunct to ERCP to detect small bile duct stones. Despite the advances in CT, EUS is still useful in patients with suspected or known pancreatic tumours. When CT scan is used alone, too many patients are subjected to laparotomy only to find that resection is not possible. The advent of EUS-guided FNA has added tremendously to the information that can be obtained from an EUS examination. Finally, EUS will probably prove to be very helpful in cases in which the clinician, perhaps to evaluate mid-epigastric pain of unknown cause, wishes to rule out chronic pancreatitis as a possible cause.

References

1. Edmundowicz SA, Aliperti G, Middleton WD. Preliminary experience using endoscopic ultrasonography in the diagnosis of choledocholithiasis. Endoscopy. 1992;24:774–8.
2. Amouyal P, Amouyal G, Levy P et al. Diagnosis of choledocholithiasis by endoscopic ultrasonography. Gastroenterology. 1994;106:1062–7.
3. Aubertin JM, Levoir D, Bouillot JL et al. Endoscopic ultrasonography immediately prior to laparoscopic cholecystectomy: a prospective evaluation. Endoscopy. 1996;28:667–73.
4. Prat F, Amouyal G, Amouyal P et al. Prospective controlled study of endoscopic ultrasonography and endoscopic retrograde cholangiography in patients with suspected common-bile duct lithiasis. Lancet. 1996;347(8994):75–9.
5. Canto MI, Chak A, Stellato T, Sivak MV Jr. Endoscopic ultrasonography versus cholangiography for the diagnosis of choledocholithiasis. Gastrointest Endosc. 1998;47:439–48.
6. Yasuda K, Nakajima M, Kawai K. Diseases of the biliary tract and papilla of Vater. In: Kawai K, ed. Endoscopic Ultrasonography in Gastroenterology. Tokyo: Igaku Shoin, 1988:96–105.
7. Tio TL, Cheng J, Wijers OB et al. Endosonographic TNM staging of extrahepatic bile duct cancer: comparison with pathologic staging. Gastroenterology. 1991;100:1351–61.
8. Mukai H, Cho V, Yasuda K et al. Evaluation of endoscopic ultrasonography in the diagnosis of cancer extension in the papilla of Vater and common bile duct. Gastrointest Endosc. 1990;36:201(abstract).
9. Mitake M, Nakazawa S, Nitoh Y et al. Endoscopic ultrasonography in diagnosis of extent of gallbladder carcinoma. Gastrointest Endosc. 1990;36:562–6.
10. Tamada K, Ido K, Ueno N et al. Preoperative staging of extrahepatic bile duct cancer with intraductal ultrasonography. Am J Gastroenterol. 1995;90:239–46.
11. Kuroiwa M, Tsukamoto Y, Mitake M et al. New techniques using intraductal ultrasonography for the diagnosis of bile duct cancer. Ultrasound Med. 1994;13:189–95.
12. Waxman I. Characterization of a malignant bile duct obstruction by intraductal ultrasonography. Am J Gastroenterol. 1995;90:1073–5.

13. Palazzo L, Roseau G, Gayet B et al. Endoscopic ultrasonography in adenocarcinoma of the pancreas. Results of a prospective study with comparison to ultrasonography and CT scan. Endoscopy. 1993;25:143–50.
14. Rosch T, Braig C, Gain T et al. Staging of pancreatic and ampullary carcinoma by endoscopic ultrasonography. Comparison with conventional ultrasonography, computed tomography and angiography. Gastroenterology. 1992;102:188–99.
15. Yasuda K, Mukai H, Fujimoto S et al. The diagnosis of pancreatic cancer by endoscopic ultrasonography. Gastrointest Endosc. 1988;34:1–8.
16. Rosch T, Lorenz R, Braig C et al. Endoscopic ultrasound in pancreatic tumor diagnosis. Gastrointest Endosc. 1991;37:347–52.
17. Tio, TL, Tytgat GNJ. Evaluation of resectability of gastrointestinal tumors. In: Kawai K, ed. Endoscopic Ultrasonography in Gastroenterology. Tokyo: Igakushoin, 1988:106–18.
18. Rosch T, Dittler HJ, Lorenz R et al. The endosonographic staging of pancreatic carcinoma. Dtsch Med Wochenschr. 1992;117:563–9.
19. Legmann P, Vignaux O, Dousset B et al. Pancreatic tumors: comparison of dual-phase helical CT and endoscopic ultrasonography. Am J Roentgenol. 1998;170:1315–22.
20. Midwinter MJ, Beveridge CJ, Wilsdon JB et al. Correlation between spiral computed tomography, endoscopic ultrasonography and findings at operation in pancreatic and ampullary tumors. Br J Surg. 1999;86:189–93.
21. Nattermann C, Goldschmidt AJ, Dancygier H. Endosonography in chronic pancreatitis – a comparison between endoscopic retrograde pancreatography and endoscopic ultrasonography (See comments). Endoscopy. 1993;25:565–70.
22. Catalano MF, Lahoti S, Geenen JE, Hogan WJ. Prospective evaluation of endoscopic ultrasonography, endoscopic retrograde pancreatography, and secretin test in the diagnosis of chronic pancreatitis. Gastrointest Endosc. 1998;48:11–17.
23. Wiersema MJ, Hawes RH, Lehman GA et al. Prospective evaluation of endoscopic ultrasonography and endoscopic retrograde cholangiopancreatography in patients with chronic abdominal pain of suspected pancreatic origin. Endoscopy. 1993;25:555–64.
24. Lees WR. Endoscopic ultrasonography of chronic pancreatitis and pancreatic pseudocysts. Scand J Gastroenterol Suppl. 1986;123:123–9.
25. Wallace MB, Hawes RH, Durkalski V et al. The reliability of endoscopic ultrasound for the diagnosis of chronic pancreatitis: interobserver agreement among experienced endosonographers. Gastrointest Endosc. 2001;53:294–9.
26. Lau JY, Sung JJ, Chan AC et al. Stigmata of hemorrhage in bleeding peptic ulcers: an interobserver agreement study among international experts. Gastrointest Endosc. 1997;46:33–6.
27. von Kummer R, Holle R, Gizyska U et al. Interobserver agreement in assessing early CT signs of middle cerebral artery infarction. Am J Neuroradiol. 1996;17:1743–8.
28. Lok CE, Morgan CD, Ranganathan N. The accuracy and interobserver agreement in detecting the 'gallop sounds' by cardiac auscultation. Chest. 1998;114:1283–8.
29. Zimmerman MJ, Mishra G, Lewin DN et al. Comparison of EUS findings with histopathology in chronic pancreatitis. Gastrointest Endosc. 1997;45:AB185(abstract).
30. Buscail L, Escourrou J, Moreau J et al. Endoscopic ultrasonography in chronic pancreatitis: a comparative prospective study with conventional ultrasonography, computed tomography, and ERCP. Pancreas. 1995;10:251–7.
31. Sahai AV, Zimmerman M, Aabakken L et al. Prospective assessment of the ability of endoscopic ultrasound to diagnose, exclude, or establish the severity of chronic pancreatitis found by endoscopic retrograde cholangiopancreatography. Gastrointest Endosc. 1998;48:18–25.
32. Raimondo M, Clain JE, Wang KK et al. Can EUS detect early or severe chronic pancreatitis (CP)? Comparison of endoscopic ultrasonography with pancreatic function. Gastroenterology. 1998;114:A492.
33. Zuccaro G, Conwell DL, Vargo JJ et al. The role of endoscopic ultrasound (EUS) in the diagnosis of early and advanced chronic pancreatitis (CP). Gastroenterology. 2000;118:A674.
34. Hastier P, Buckley MJ, Francois E et al. A prospective study of pancreatic disease in patients with alcoholic cirrhosis: comparative diagnostic value of ERCP and EUS and long-term significance of isolated parenchymal abnormalities. Gastrointest Endosc. 1999;49:705–9.
35. Bhutani MS. Endoscopic ultrasonography: changes of chronic pancreatitis in asymptomatic and symptomatic alcoholic patients. J Ultrasound Med. 1999;18:455–62.

Section III
Procedure and perception

6
What is the time required for a good endoscopy? Time for training

G. A. LEHMAN

Appropriate training for the next generation of endoscopists is a mandatory task. Many first-generation endoscopists were self-taught, but this is no longer acceptable. Gastrointestinal endoscopy training should occur in a setting which offers comprehensive study of gastrointestinal diseases. Endoscopy societies from Australia and the United States of America have published similar minimal standards/guidelines requiring hands-on training of 125–150 upper endoscopies (with or without biopsy) and 150–200 colonoscopies (with or without biopsy) exams. The time required to accomplish this training can be years (overall training) but this report will focus on time/individual exams.

Many factors affect training time and the teaching process. Endoscopes with smaller diameters (7–10 mm) are generally well tolerated, but 5–6 mm diameter endoscopes are more difficult to use, especially for trainees. Performance of unsedated exams is more common, but deeper sedation, as with propofol, is gaining use, especially for colonoscopy. The instructor is fully legally responsible for the examination. Government payers (in the USA) require that the instructor be present to view the entire exam.

Worldwide, the utilization of gastrointestinal endoscopy continues to grow as barium studies decrease and use in screening studies, such as for colorectal cancer, increases. This makes more teaching exams available. Decreasing reimbursement per case is occurring in the USA; therefore motivating more rapid endoscopy and room turnover to maintain stable income. Video endoscopic systems facilitate the teaching process and training. Simulators for endoscopic training are available and improving in quality, but remain costly. There are limited data showing improved sigmoidoscopy skill levels after simulator practice. Reports may be written, dictated or computer program-generated. The above factors may result in total room time of 15–20 minutes for upper gastrointestinal endoscopy and 15–30 minutes for colonoscopy. There are no data on the correct time allotments for teaching. In our own method in early stages of training (up to 25–50 exams), trainees will be given hands-on time of 5–10 minutes per case and require an almost-complete re-do of the entire exam by the instructor. Later the trainee will be allowed 5–20 minutes per exam and only verbal instruction/discussion may be needed. As skill develops, more complex tasks (gastrointestinal bleed therapy, polypectomy, etc.) can be added, still within the same time limit. Training can (should) continue when the instructor is 'driving' with discussions of technique, pathophysiology or patient management. Generally the trainee is required to generate the first draft of the report.

Over the course of a 2–3-year training interval the trainees initially appear to be costly and money/time-expensive[1]. Later they appear to improve in efficiency as they facilitate consultations, obtain informed consents and generate procedure reports. Overall, I believe trainees are cost/time neutral.

Reference

1. McCashland T, Brand R, Lyden E, de Garmo P, and CORI Research Project. The time and financial impact of training fellows in endoscopy. Am J Gastroenterol. 2000;95:3129–32.

7
Improved gastrointestinal imaging – improved outcome for patients?

S. HOLLERBACH

DETECTION OF PRECANCEROUS LESIONS AND EARLY CANCER IN THE GASTROINTESTINAL (GI) TRACT

The clinical outcome of advanced GI malignancies such as oesophageal squamous cell carcinoma and adenocarcinoma located in the oesophagus, stomach, small bowel, and colorectum, is still poor[1-3]. Upon establishment of a definite cancer diagnosis the 5-year relative survival rate is only 4% for oesophageal cancer[1,2], 12% for gastric cancer[3], and around 40% for colorectal cancer. In contrast, lesions detected at an early stage, such as high-grade dysplasia (= intraepithelial neoplasia) and T1 carcinoma (confined to mucosa/superficial submucosa) are associated with an excellent long-term prognosis. The 5-year survival rate for early stomach cancer exceeds 90%[4,5], for early colonic cancer it is in excess of 97%[6], and for superficial squamous T1 stage oesophageal cancers the 5-year survival compares favourably around 83%[7]. In this context early and superficial cancers of the oesophagus, stomach, and colon denote carcinomas confined to the mucosal and/or superficial submucosal layers, regardless of any regional lymph node involvement[7-13]. Hence there is a tremendous clinical need in Western countries such as Germany and the US to improve GI imaging for the detection of premalignant, precancerous and early lesions such as high-grade dysplasia and T1 carcinoma lesions that can be located in all parts of the GI tract and surrounding tissues. The overall prognosis of early malignancies largely depends on the extent of local submucosal and local lymphatic invasion (lymphatic spread, L stage) which has been known for many years[7-13]. Techniques that can disclose even small cancerous GI lesions are based solely on endoscopic and endosonographic techniques. At present no invasive ('virtual' computerized tomography (CT) imaging, positron emission tomography (PET) scan) or non-invasive external imaging modality such as abdominal high-end ultrasound (US) or magnetic resonance tomography (MRI) are deemed likely to ever permit sufficient resolution of specific GI structures such as mucosal surfaces and the bowel wall to detect small curable lesions. Hence, diagnostic strategies to first detect premalignant lesions (high-grade dysplasia) at a curative stage in precancerous settings such as Barrett's oesophagus, HNPCC, familial polyposis syndromes (FAP), and others, must focus on further improvements of endoscopic techniques.

There are several putative reasons why Western endoscopists have been relatively unsuccessful in detecting early cancers. In Japan most early cancers are found sporadically by a meticulous use of endoscopic techniques, and only 10% of gastric cancers are disclosed by occupational screening programmes[14]. In addition, Japanese investigators routinely use dye spraying to examine minute and subtle mucosal abnormalities such as flat intramucosal polyps or 'dysplasia-associated lesion or mass' (DALM) in ulcerative colitis that carry a clear risk of early cancer upon detection. One old technique (chromoendoscopy) and several new endoscopic techniques (zoom endoscopy, autofluorescence, light-induced fluorescence endoscopy, photodynamic diagnosis, optical coherence tomography (OCT), confocal laser microscopy, light-scattering spectroscopy and others) have recently been developed and are currently undergoing clinical trials to assess their ability to detect even small early precancerous and malignant lesions, and to evaluate their potential clinical role in this setting.

All techniques to detect dysplasia and early cancers in the GI tract have one thing in common: circumscript or diffusely scattered dysplastic lesions or early T1 cancers confined to the mucosa and/or superficial submucosa (T1m, sm) that are found during such procedures can eventually be subjected to definite endoscopic (endoscopic mucosal resection; EMR, photodynamic therapy) or surgical treatment. Endoscopic treatment frequently takes place within the same session, and preliminary studies suggest that the clinical outcome of EMR is readily comparable to standard operative procedures, while being far less invasive[20].

IMPROVED IMAGING TECHNIQUES FOR THE GI TRACT

Chromoendoscopy

Among these techniques, chromoendoscopy, which has been used in Japan for decades, has re-emerged to improve the detection of early lesions in the oesophagus, stomach, and colon also in Western populations[14]. Preliminary studies show promising results, particularly regarding improvement in the detection of high-grade dysplasia in Barrett's oesophagus, though the full potential of the technique may first emerge in combination with magnifying endoscopy, which is presently undergoing extensive scientific evaluation. Dye spraying techniques have the great advantage of being relatively simple, cheap, fast, and widely available, and they can be easily combined with other modalities such as zoom endoscopes and high-frequency ultrasound miniprobes (EUS). *Methylene blue* is used to identify areas of *Barrett's* intestinal metaplasia[15-18], which may help in targeting biopsies so as to disclose intraepithelial neoplasia (dysplasia)[16]. However, it is still controversial to what extent methylene blue staining is really superior to standard four-quadrant biopsies and can improve detection of dysplasia and T1 cancer in clinical practice[16-18], but several ongoing studies will shortly elucidate this issue further. *Lugol's* iodine dye (0.5–5%) binds to glycogen-rich epithelial cells and thus stains the normal oesophageal squamous epithelium brown or greenish, while areas of intraepithelial neoplasia remain unstained[19]. Examples of methylene blue staining and Lugol's staing are demonstrated in Figures 1 and 2. Indigo

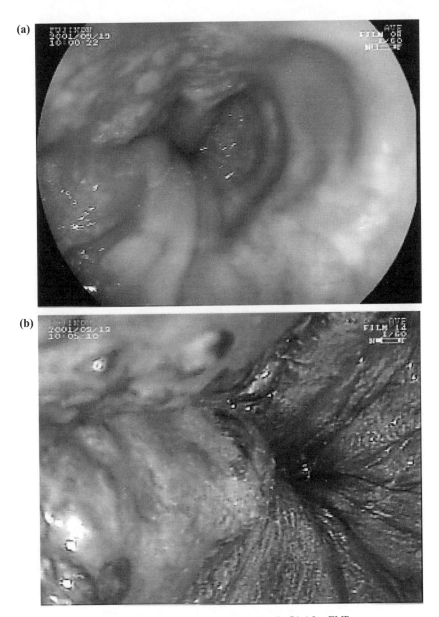

Figure 1 Lugol's solution (5%) **(a)** Barnett's mucosa (stained); **(b)** After EMR

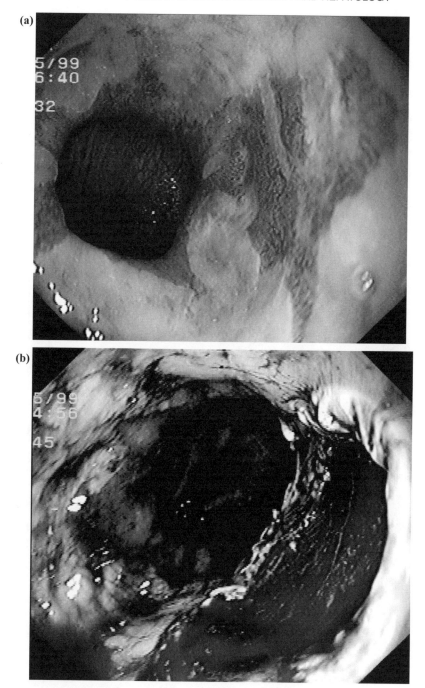

Figure 2 Methylene blue (1%) **(a)** Barnett's mucosa (stained); **(b)** After EMR

carmine dye (0.2%) staining is useful to highlight suspicious mucosal irregularities both in the stomach and colon, since this dye accentuates mucosal surface contours and hence defines the margins of elevated and flat lesions (Figure 3). Other dye stains are India ink, cresyl violet, phenol red, toluidine blue, and Congo red, whose diagnostic potential is probably limited to special indications and selected patients. Outcome studies, however, that clearly demonstrate that dye spraying detects dysplasia and early cancer more accurately than biopsy techniques, or that use of chromoendoscopy significantly affects morbidity, mortality, survival, or the overall clinical course of the patients, are still lacking.

Other experimental techniques (induced fluorescence, autofluorescence, magnifying endoscopy, optical coherence tomography, optical biopsy, light-scattering spectroscopy)

Other endoscopic techniques to detect (pre-)malignant lesions, however, have been newly developed. The following procedures have been developed to further facilitate surface detection and assessment of the depth of tumour invasion even of very tiny lesions in suspicious areas found with high-resolution-endoscopy or chromoendoscopy. Several different physical approaches such as optical surface magnification techniques ('zoom endoscopy'), light dispersion or scattering modes, OCT, photodynamic diagnosis by induced fluorescence (PDT) and autofluorescence of tissues, and 'virtual optical biopsies' by using endoscopic confocal laser microscopy are currently undergoing extensive scientific and clinical investigation, particularly in Japan. While all these techniques may further improve detection and invasion of limited malignancies in the GI tract, clinical studies first have to establish whether each new procedure has a potential clinical role in this setting that clearly justifies the cost, workload, and particularly the side-effects associated with systemic exposure to medical agents such as 5-aminolevulinic acid (5-ALA) for PDT. Though clinical outcome studies are still lacking, the near future will show which of these technique(s) besides chromoendoscopy can be recommended for standard clinical use, and how great the potential benefit for patients will be. For the small bowel, however, the novel M_2A-video-capsule endoscopy may become very useful for the detection of premalignant adenomas such as those seen in patients with familial adenomatous polyposis (Fig. 4) or FAP.

Photodynamic diagnosis (PDT)

PDT, with systemically applied exogenous substances (fluorophores) such as haematoporphyrins (5-ALA) is used to photosensitize dysplastic or neoplastic cells in patients with high risk of cancer such as Barrett's oesophagus and ulcerative colitis. Metabolic fluorophores such as protoporphyrin IX concentrate preferentially in neoplastic tissue; hence PDT can sensitively detect dysplasia in Barrett's oesophagus[21] and other premalignant conditions such as dysplastic gastric adenoma. Other fluorophores include flavoproteins, structural proteins, and cytosolic granules of eosinophils. Photosensitized dysplastic tissues exhibit an enhanced metabolic uptake of the haematoporphyrin 5-ALA, and the resulting increase in fluorescence can be detected by the endoscopic, near-ultraviolet blue-light mode which excites the fluorophore. Biopsies can then be directed to suspicious areas that appear as red fluorescence, thereby permitting an increased

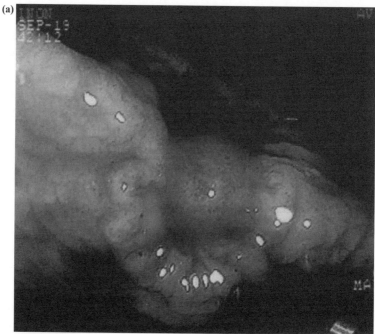

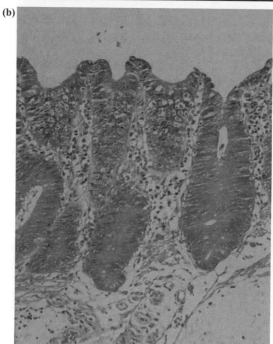

Figure 3 Ulcerative colitis. **(a)** DALM – chromoendoscopy: indigo carmine (0.4%); **(b)** Intraepithelial neoplasia

detection rate of dysplastic or neoplastic tissues. A recent clinical study[21] shows that high-grade dysplasia and superficial adenocarcinoma can be sensitively detected by systemic application of 5-ALA and endoscopic blue-light detection, but inflammatory conditions result in a very limited specificity of findings. Topical application of the fluorophore, however, is non-toxic and may enhance the yield of undirected standard biopsies in this setting, but this has to be confirmed in prospective clinical studies. Unfortunately, due to the problems with the specificity of findings and toxicity of agents, the procedure should still be considered as investigational at present.

Light-induced fluorescence (LIF) or autofluorescence (LIFE-GI) endoscopy[22]

This system uses laser-induced point fluorescence spectroscopy, which measures the differences in the remitted wavelength of dysplastic or neoplastic tissues when compared with normal tissues. Once excited to a higher energy state there is a high probability that endogenous chromophores such as water, haemoglobin, melanin, structural proteins, and others, will return or decay to their original energy state. The added energy can subsequently be re-emitted as another photon or heat up the surrounding tissue. Fluorescence is one mechanism of that photon remission, and when endogenous (or exogenous, see above) fluorophores are being excited to a higher energy state by an incident photon and then decay to a lower or ground state, energy is emitted as another photon that can be picked up by specialized measuring systems. For each fluorophore the spectrum of the fluorescence (emitted light) is unique, and the emitted light will always be of a longer wavelength than that of the emitted light. Hence, by exciting tissue at appropriate wavelengths and monitoring the emission of constituent fluorophores, it is possible to obtain information about the presence and concentrations of these substances in different tissues such as non-dysplastic mucosa and highly dysplastic Barrett's mucosa. This technique combined with endoscopy is known as LIF or autofluorescence in the gastrointestinal tract. To obtain a tissue spectrum the endoscopist touches the target with a specialized catheter probe so that light is evenly distributed over a relatively small tissue target. A fixed geometric relationship, however, between light and tissue cannot be maintained in an LIF imaging system.

Initial *in vitro* and *in vivo* studies with colonic polyps and oesophageal carcinoma approximate that of histopathological assessment[23,24]. The sensitivity, specificity, and positive predictive value reported are in the ranges 80–100%, 77–95%, and 82–94%, respectively. Despite these encouraging initial experiences, enthusiasm for LIF has been tempered by the fact that differences in fluorescence between various types of tissues are based on the architecture of the tissue and factors such as the metabolic state and light-scattering properties of each tissue layer. Hence, tissue fluorescence is complex in reality, and special characteristics that differentiate between normal layers, unspecific mucosal/submucosal abnormalities, inflammation, scarring, and dysplasia are very difficult to define. Another obvious limitation of LIF is that it is point-specific, and a tissue spectrum obtained with a probe represents only a tiny volume of tissue, thereby limiting its usefulness for surveillance purposes. Since the randomness of dysplasia in most premalignant conditions is the same for both random biopsies and sophisticated techniques such as LIF, it remains to be shown whether new developments will justify the high cost of these experimental devices, and whether LIF-based systems will ever make it into clinical practice.

Another real-time imaging system based on the principle of ratio fluorescence imaging (RFI) has been developed for the GI tract (LIFE-GI system; Xillix Technologies, Canada). Two cameras are attached to the fibre endoscope for detection of red and green fluorescence. Using this system, normal mucosa is believed to appear green, whereas dysplastic or neoplastic tissues appear red[25]. Preliminary clinical studies reported that LIFE-GI can detect early dysplastic and neoplastic lesions somewhat more sensitively than conventional sample techniques, particularly in Barrett's oesophagus and the stomach, with accuracy figures ranging between 88% and 96% upon comparison with histology[25,28]. Other studies and experience derived from studies performed in the respiratory tract, however, clearly suggest numerous diagnostic problems due to a high rate of false-positive findings that are caused by inflammation and normal Barrett's epithelium that tend to yield a red fluorescence that is difficult to distinguish from dysplasia or cancer.

Although an interesting and challenging concept, numerous 'real-life' problems such as geometry problems and a different contact of the probe and the target lesion due to movements distinctly limit the use of fluorescence imaging systems in humans. At present no clinical study has confirmed that the slightly advantageous detection rate of dysplasia and early cancer justify the high cost and level of expertise that are necessary to use such techniques in clinical standard practice.

Magnifying endoscopy (zoom)

Contrast-enhancing dyes are often used together with magnifying endoscopes that have been developed since the first introduction of flexible instruments in the late 1960s. Most instruments use an assembly that allows the position of a system of different lenses at the distal end of the fibreoptic or video scope to be changed by the endoscopist. These lenses can magnify images by ranging from 30× to 170×. As magnification increases, however, the endoscopic field becomes smaller and the slightest movement of the instrument or the target will cause a blurring of images. In combination with surface-enhancing dye spraying (indigo carmine, cresyl violet) and a significant expertise, the probability that early cancer is present within the smallest irregularity of the mucosa, its depth of invasion, and consequently the most appropriate therapy (endoscopic or surgical) can be determined[26]. With a contrast-enhancing dye and magnification, the mucosal surface of the colon appears as a pattern of numerous pits that are actually the openings at the mucosal surface of the crypts of Lieberkühn. These can be identified only by using a specialized magnifying (zoom) endoscope. Recently, the 'pit pattern' classification of normal and aberrant crypt foci by Kudo[27], which recognizes five distinct types, has been widely accepted in clinical endoscopy. Analysis of the pit pattern, together with other endoscopic observations (elevated or depressed lesion, polyp), shows a relatively close correlation to the actual histological features. Thus, it appears likely that an 'on-site' assessment of lesions ranging from benign to malignant changes can be accurately made in the near future[26], but further studies are warranted to particularly show

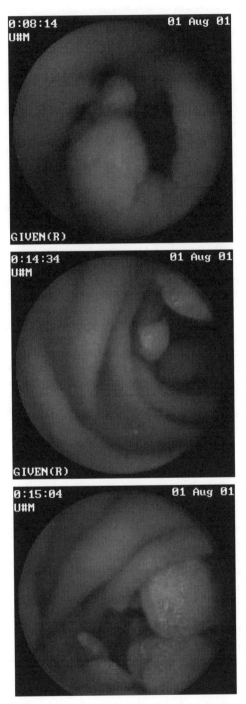

Figure 4 Small bowel precancerous lesions: video capsule (M2A) imaging of villous adenomas in FAP patients

that this time-consuming and expert approach really will pay off in an increasing number of early cancers found during routine endoscopy.

Optical coherence tomography (OCT)

OCT is an imaging modality for cross-sectional, subsurface imaging of biological tissues with high spatial resolution[29]. OCT is based on the measurement of singly backscattered light as a function of depth for image acquisition, but has been compared with B-mode ultrasound. Because OCT is an optical imaging technique, it can achieve spatial resolutions as small as 4–10 μm which is 10–25× greater than the resolution obtained with high-frequency endoscopic ultrasound (EUS), MRI, and CT. However, the depth of imaging of OCT is limited to approximately 2–3 mm, which excludes accurate T- and particularly N-staging of cancerous lesions. When compared with EUS, OCT not only images the GI wall layers, but also assesses structure and potentially cellular features. Different tissues have different light reflectance properties[30], and the images are based on the reflectance of cell membranes, collagen, adipose tissue, muscle tissue, etc. The interferometric information gathered can be transferred to a detector and demodulator, transformed into polar images, and finally converted into coloured images on a computer screen[31]. Since 1997 several studies with OCT have been performed in humans[31,32]. Preliminary studies showed that OCT in humans is feasible and safe, and all wall layers of the normal oesophageal wall were visible with a complete loss of the layer structure in carcinomatous lesions. Advances in OCT imaging techniques made it possible to visualize the entire lumen of intestinal hollow organs by providing a 360-degree real-time OCT image. Such instruments provide high-resolution images of tiny areas of the mucosal surfaces, and the technique apparently works best in the oesophagus and colon[31]. Preliminary correlation studies *in vitro* show that OCT images can be almost equivalent to microscopic sections of the wall layers, thus providing 'semi-histological', in-depth images of the wall structure in the GI tract. Thus, OCT has the highest resolution of all techniques currently in use, which makes it a very attractive candidate for deciding whether or not EMR can be safely applied. Preliminary clinical studies suggest that OCT might be of benefit in premalignant conditions characterized by mucosal transitions from low-grade dysplasia to invasive carcinoma, especially premalignant conditions in which this transition is difficult to detect by standard endoscopy. Pilot studies in patients with Barrett's oesophagus indicate that normal squamous epithelium and Barrett's metaplasia can be readily differentiated by OCT[33]. A characteristic difference may be the loss of the layered structure of the squamous epithelium. In addition, these are changes in the appearance of cellularity, gland structure, and brightness of the different wall layers. Thus, OCT appears attractive in the assessment of early cancer before, and after, local tumour ablation such as EMR is applied.

The practical depth of OCT imaging is at present limited to 1–3 mm, which can be a major disadvantage, particularly in submucosal lesions. Other problems of OCT include the lack of convincing evidence suggesting that dysplastic mucosa indeed scatters light in a different way than non-dysplastic and inflamed (or scarred) tissue. Furthermore, the application to cellular layers at present lacks clinical feasibility and utility, while it remains to be seen whether OCT can detect dysplastic mucosa even in the absence of clues to its presence by standard endoscopic observation. In summary, OCT as applied to endoscopy is a rather immature technology, and ongoing studies within the near future will show whether further technical modifications such as Doppler OCT will become a clinically useful adjunct to high-resolution video endoscopy.

Other imaging techniques

EUS, performed with small 'through-the-scope' ultrasound miniprobes and frequencies between 12.5 and 20 mHz, permits the endoscopist to rapidly gain an overview over up to 12 different wall layers in the GI tract. This technique is very useful in lesions that are detected during high-resolution endoscopy and confirmed histologically to consist of precancerous or cancerous tissue. EUS miniprobes can then be used to differentiate between mucosal ($T1_m$) and submucosal ($T1_{sm}$) invasion of the cancerous lesion. Hence, EUS results have a reasonable accuracy for the local (T- and N-) staging of early cancer, and facilitate the application of local endoscopic resection techniques in selected patients, while the decision for a combined laparoscopic/endoscopic or surgical resection can be based on EUS miniprobe results. However, since EUS does not replace histology, and tends to overestimate the invasion depths of some cancers, its ability to predict the outcome of the resection technique appears to be limited at present, and further outcome studies must elucidate its role in future clinical practice.

Imaging dysplasia at a microscopic level during endoscopy is called *optical biopsy*. Confocal laser microscopy is being combined with standard endoscopic observation of tissue points, which has been shown to be feasible under experimental *in vitro* conditions and in experimental animals. The near future will show whether this technique is useful to increase the yield of early cancers found; it may also eventually result in a gain of clinically relevant information that justifies the high cost of the equipment.

Other new techniques are *light-scattering spectroscopy* and *Raman spectroscopy* that have recently been reviewed elsewhere[34]. Raman spectroscopy is based on changes induced by light in the vibrational and rotational states of molecular bonds. When emitted photons cause the electron cloud of a molecule to oscillate, some of the energy may transfer to the molecule, exciting it to a higher vibrational state. As a result of this interaction a photon of longer wavelength will be re-emitted, a phenomenon known as Raman scattering. Raman imaging has the potential to detect changes in cells and tissues before they result in gross or even histological changes. Promising results have been obtained under experimental conditions using the full range of possible interactions of light and tissue, including scattering and Raman scattering. Though Raman scattering looks extremely attractive because of its specificity, the complexities of a true Raman imaging system are daunting, and further studies will first have to concentrate on these difficult technical questions.

SUMMARY AND DISCUSSION

A tremendous effort is necessary to reduce mortality rates for digestive tract cancer through the use of endoscopy and other techniques. At present it appears to be the best strategy to identify precursor lesions such as dysplasia and intraepithelial neoplasms in high-risk patients in its earliest stages. The best techniques currently available are advanced endoscopic equipment in combination with ancillary techniques to gain more information concerning the extent and penetration depth of lesions found during the same clinical procedure. For some disorders, such as colorectal cancer, the precursor lesions (polyps) are readily evident at routine endoscopy; while in other disorders, such as Barrett's oesophagus or long-standing ulcerative colitis, the precursor lesions are frequently elusive, and standard endoscopic imaging is not sufficient. For these considerations several new ancillary imaging techniques are needed to move beyond simple observation, and the techniques reviewed above represent just an array of possible procedures to fulfil this task. To a large extent, efforts to improve the endoscopic detection of dysplastic mucosa and early-stage cancer derive from the interactions of ultrasound and light with tissue. The available techniques are based on two principal approaches: imaging dysplasia at the microscopic level, and identification of biochemical indicators of dysplasia. Promising results have been obtained under experimental conditions, using the full range of possible interactions such as light scattering, photodynamic diagnosis, EUS, autofluorescence, and Raman scattering. However, the transition to practical imaging systems that provide incremental information with relevant clinical information is more difficult. So far, monitoring of light–tissue interactions with catheter probes and fluorescence techniques is only marginally better than random biopsy approaches, but the actual gain in terms of patient care is most likely insufficient to warrant acquisition of such expensive systems by the practising endoscopist. It is very difficult to forecast which one(s) of the various techniques to improve detection of precancerous lesions will prove so useful that it is extended into clinical practice. Magnifying endoscopy in combination with chromoendoscopic surface contour enhancement dyes appears very attractive, and the combination with OCT or EUS may provide all sufficient local information concerning early cancer lesions needed for clinical purposes. OCT alone is also promising since it provides actual images of tissue layers. However, the ability to image larger tissue surface areas efficiently and rapidly is problematic. Of the various interactions between light and tissue, LIF spectroscopy is the best-studied entity, but results obtained with catheter probes appear to be difficult to duplicate with a LIF imaging system. It is very likely that the growing body of knowledge regarding the fundamental physics of light–tissue interaction known as light scattering will result in the development of even more advanced imaging systems in the near future. In the meantime, inexpensive and easy techniques such as chromoendoscopy should be used much more widely, especially in Western countries.

References

1. Earlam R, Cunha-Melo JR. Oesophageal squamous cell carcinoma: I. A critical review of surgery. Br J Surg. 1980;67:381–90.
2. Earlam R, Cunha-Melo JR. Oesophageal squamous cell carcinoma: II. A critical review of radiotherapy. Br J Surg. 1980;67:391–7.
3. Everett SM, Axon ATR. Early gastric cancer: disease or pseudo-disease. Lancet. 1998;351: 1350–2.

4. Sue-Ling HM, Martin I, Griffith J et al. Early gastric cancer: 46 cases in one surgical department. Gut. 1992;33:1318–22.
5. Yamazaki H, Oshima A, Murakami R. A long-term follow-up study of patients with gastric cancer detected by mass screening. Cancer. 1989;63:613–17.
6. Moreaux J, Catala M. Carcinoma of the colon: long-term survival and prognosis after surgical treatment in a series of 798 patients. World J Surg. 1987;11:804–9.
7. Kato H, Tachimori Y, Watanabe H et al. Superficial oesophageal carcinoma. Surgical treatment and the results. Cancer. 1990;66: 2319–23.
8. Endo M, Yoshino K, Takeshita K et al. Analysis of 1125 cases of early oesophageal carcinoma in Japan. Dis Oesophagus. 1991;2:71–6.
9. Tajima Y, Nakanishi Y, Tachimori Y et al. Histopathologic findings predicting lymph node metastases and prognosis of patients with superficial esophageal carcinoma. Cancer. 2000; 88:1285–93.
10. Moreaux J, Bougaran J. Early gastric cancer. A 25-year surgical experience. Ann Surg. 1993; 217:347–55.
11. Perri F, Iuliano R, Valente G et al. Minute and small early gastric cancers in a Western population: a clinicopathologic study on 80 cases. Dig Dis Sci. 1995;41:475–80.
12. Baba H, Maehara Y, Okuyama T et al. Lymph node metastases and macroscopic features in early gastric cancer. Hepatogastroenterology. 1994;41:380–3.
13. Meahara Y, Orita H, Okuyama T et al. Predictors of lymph node metastasis in early gastric cancer. Br J Surg. 1992;79:245–7.
14. Rembacken BJ, Gotoda T, Fujii T, Axon ATR. Endoscopic mucosal resection. Endoscopy. 2001;33:709–18.
15. Fennerty MB, Sampliner RE, McGee D et al. Intestinal metaplasia of the oesophagus. Identification by a selective mucosal staining technique. Gastrointest Endosc. 1992;38:696–8.
16. Canto MIF, Setrakian S, Willis J et al. Methylene blue-directed biopsies improve detection of intestinal metaplasia and dysplasia in Barrett's oesophagus. Gastrointest Endosc. 2000; 51:560–8.
17. Wo JM, Ray MB, Mayfield-Stokes S et al. Comparison of methylene blue-directed biopsies and conventional biopsies in the detection of intestinal metaplasia and dysplasia in Barrett's oesophagus: a preliminary study. Gastrointest Endosc. 2001;54:294–301.
18. Sharma P, Topalovski M, Mayo MS, Weston AP. Methylene blue chromoendoscopy for detection of short-segment Barrett's oesophagus. Gastrointest Endosc. 2001;54:289–93.
19. Misumi A, Harada K, Muratami A. Role of Lugol's dye endoscopy in the diagnosis of early oesophageal cancer. Endoscopy. 1990;22:12–16.
20. Ell C, May A, Gossner L et al. Endoscopic mucosal resection of early cancer and high-grade dysplasia in Barrett's oesophagus. Gastroenterology. 2000;118:670–7.
21. Endlicher E, Knüchel R, Hauser T, Szeimies RM, Schölmerich J, Messmann H. Endoscopic fluorescence detection of low and high grade dysplasia in Barrett's oesophagus using systemic or local 5-aminolaevulinic acid sensitization. Gut. 2001;48:314–9.
22. Richards-Kortum R, Rava R, Petras RE, Fitzmaurice M, Sivak M, Feld M. Spectroscopic diagnosis of colonic dysplasia. Photochem Photobiol. 1991;53:777–86.
23. Haringsma L, Tytgat GN. The value of fluorescence techniques in gastrointestinal endoscopy. Better than the endoscopist's eye? I: The European experience. Endoscopy. 1998;30:416–18.
24. Wang TD, Van Dam J, Crawford JM, Presinger EA, Wang Y, Feld MS. Fluorescence endoscopic imaging of human colonic adenomas. Gastroenterology. 1996;111:1182–91.
25. Duvall GA, Saidi R, Kost J et al. Real-time light induced fluorescence endoscopy in the gastrointestinal tract. Gastrointest Endosc. 1997;45:AB28.
26. Saitoh Y, Obara T, Watari J et al. Invasion depth diagnosis of depressed type early colorectal cancers by combined use of videoendoscopy and chromoendoscopy. Gastrointest Endosc. 1998;48:362–70.
27. Kudo S. Early colorectal cancer and endoscopic resection. In: Sivak MV Jr, ed. Gastroenterologic Endoscopy, 2nd edn. Philadelphia: Saunders, 2000:262–71.
28. Abe S, Izuishi K, Tajiri H, Kinoshita T, Matsuoka T. Correlation of *in vitro* autofluorescence endoscopy images with histopathologic findings in stomach cancer. Endoscopy. 2000;32:281–6.
29. Huang D, Swanson EA, Lin CP et al. Optical coherence tomography. Science. 1991;254:1178–81.
30. Tadrous PJ. Methods for imaging the structure and function of living tissues and cells: I. Optical coherence tomography. J Pathol. 2000;191:115–19.

31. Sivak MV, Kobayashi K, Izatt JA *et al*. High-resolution endoscopic imaging of the GI tract using optical coherence tomography. Gastrointest Endosc. 2000;51:474–9.
32. Sergeev AM, Gelikonov VM, Gelikonov GV, Feldchtein FI, Kuranov RV, Gladkova ND. *In vivo* endoscopic OCT imaging of precancer and cancer states of human mucosa. Optics Express. 1997;1:432–40.
33. Seitz U: *In vivo* endoscopic optical coherence tomography of oesophagitis, Barrett's oesophagus, and adenocarcinoma of the oesophagus. Gastrointest Endosc. 2000;51:AB93.
34. Pfau PR, Sivak MV Jr. Endoscopic diagnostics. Gastroenterology. 2001;120:763–81.

8
What does the surgeon expect from preoperative imaging in liver tumours?

T. BECKER, H. S. B. FRERICKS, F. LEHNER, R. LÜCK,
H. BEKTAS, B. NASHAN, M. GALANSKI and J. KLEMPNAUER

INTRODUCTION

The liver is often the seat of primary and secondary liver tumours and, for many gastrointestinal tumours, is the site of primary metastasis. Isolated organ infiltration can often be found without any evidence of extrahepatic metastases. For most primary and secondary liver tumours, modern radical surgical treatment so far represents the only curative therapeutic option. In this connection, the achievement of a so-called RO resection, i.e. the *en-bloc* removal of the tumour with a sufficient margin of safety, is the most important prognostic factor[1-5]. The technical possibility of resection is dependent on the size of the tumour, the number of tumour nodes and the tumour location. A better understanding of the anatomical and physiological principles, in particular segment anatomy and the regenerative capability of the liver, as well as diagnostic, anaesthesiological and surgical technical advances have, in the last few years, led to an increase in resectioning interventions with increasingly good results. The introduction of extracorporeal operating techniques (*ex-situ, in-situ, ante-situ*) in cases with badly located tumours in the porta of the liver or in the hepatic venous confluence has also increased the spectrum of resection possibilities[6,7].

In addition to malignant tumours, the development of modern diagnostic processes also enables benign liver tumours to be detected and characterized. Clinically, the most important representatives of these benign liver tumours are focal nodular hyperplasia (FNH), liver haemangioma and liver cell adenoma; these will also be dealt with briefly below.

With so many diagnostic procedures for imaging liver lesions, diagnostics must be deployed, in each individual case, in a focussed and well-considered way with respect to the clinical problem, avoiding untargeted applications.

The diagnostics used should be up-to-date, cost-effective, have low risks for the patient and also be as specific and sensitive as possible.

GENERAL ASPECTS OF THE PREOPERATIVE DIAGNOSIS OF LIVER TUMOURS

Preoperative diagnostics of liver tumours, besides generally clarifying the possibility of operating, are also used to estimate liver function and functional hepatic parenchymal reserve, as well as ascertaining intrahepatic tumour extent and excluding distant metastases (see Table 1). These aspects are of significance for decisions about further tactical procedures. It must further be considered that liver function can be negatively affected by fatty liver, cholestasis, cholangitis, prior damage due to alcohol, or past chemotherapy. Whilst, in a healthy liver, extensive resections with only 25–30% residual parenchyma can be sufficient to maintain liver function, even locally limited resections in advanced liver cirrhosis can lead to decompensated liver function[8]. For a better estimation of the residual liver volume, volumetry can be used based on modern tomographic procedures by the deployment of post-processing systems. This makes it possible to determine the volumes of the whole liver and the liver segment as well as the tumours. In addition, positional relationships can be displayed in three dimensions (3D) and shown interactively to the surgeon[9]. Liver volumetry has clinical relevance in liver donation for transplants, in cases of special tumour locations in the porta of the liver or in the hepatic venous star, in which special operating procedures are taken into consideration. In sum, preoperative diagnostics should have evaluated the findings as precisely as possible in order to avoid unnecessary laparotomies. However, in spite of all the diagnostic and laboratory chemical methods available, situations will remain in which an explorative laparotomy is necessary for definitive clarification. Independently of all diagnostic advances, the macroscopic intraoperative assessment of the liver by an operator skilled in liver surgery is also of great importance for an overall assessment of the findings with respect to consistency, parenchymal quality, and the possibility of resection.

Table 1 Results of preoperative diagnostics before surgical liver intervention

1. Exclusion/confirmation of a tumour finding
2. Type of tumour
   Benign/malignant lesions?
   Metastasis or primary liver tumour?
3. Extent of tumour
   Number, size, position
   Infiltration of vessels, central bile ducts, hepatic veins
4. Functional residual parenchyma
   Volume of the residual parenchyma
   Cirrhosis, ascites, cholestasis
5. Extrahepatic tumour
   Distant metastases, regional lymph node metastases

PREOPERATIVE DIAGNOSTICS IN PRIMARY MALIGNANT TUMOURS OF THE LIVER

Hepatocellular carcinoma

Hepatocellular carcinoma (HCC) is the most frequent liver tumour, occuring in 84% of malignant liver tumours, and is the seventh most frequent tumour worldwide. In Europe, it accounts for 4% of all malignant tumours[10]. HCC arises in 80–90% of cases on a foundation of liver cirrhosis and only develops exceptionally in a healthy liver[11,12]. Liver resection in advanced cirrhosis is frequently impossible, even in the case of small tumours: only 20–30% of patients with an HCC in cirrhosis appear to be resectable[12]. The high recurrence rate after resection, up to 60% even after oncologically adequate resection, and the 5-year survival rate of only 17% demonstrate the problem of the multifocality of HCC in cirrhosis and the carcinogenic potential of cirrhosis[13]. The multifocal nature of HCC in cirrhosis can make precise tumour staging difficult, particularly distinguishing between a highly differentiated HCC and a regenerate node. Therefore, reliable information on intrahepatic tumour spread and extrahepatic tumour manifestation is decisive for an resection treatment or liver transplant. If, in the case of a patient with an HCC in cirrhosis, a liver transplant is being considered, the diagnosis should be able to make clear statements about established prognostic criteria. Favourable prognostic factors in which a liver transplant can be considered are: solitary tumour, size <5 cm, less than three tumour nodes, no vascular invasion and no extrahepatic tumour manifestations. A positive lymph node infestation or tumour invasion into the main branches of the portal vein is associated with a significantly worse survival rate[14–18]. A positive lymph node infestation is rare in tumours smaller than 5 cm: in patients who had a liver transplant for an HCC smaller than 5 cm, positive lymph nodes could be ascertained in only 6%[22]. Tumour recurrence is markedly higher in cases with vascular invasion than those without vascular invasion (73% compared with 29%)[14] and, whilst extrahepatic tumour infestation can be predicted with comparative certainty by means of modern tomographic diagnosis, difficulties still exist in the differentiation of existing from non-existent vascular infiltration. Only with careful selection and taking into consideration these prognostic criteria can a 5-year survival of around 75% be achieved after liver transplantation. This is similar to the survival rates in benign basic disease[19–23].

Cholangiocellular carcinoma

Cholangiocellular carcinoma (CCC) is an adenocarcinoma beginning in the intrahepatic bile duct epithelium; in contrast to HCC, it does not usually develop in the cirrhotic liver. Older patients are more frequently affected, and men more than women. The risk factors for development of CCC are: thorotrast applications, and congenital cystic anomalies of the bile ducts in which serious recidivating inflammation with stone formation occur, e.g. the Caroli syndrome or primary sclerosing cholangitis (PSC) which plays an important role in Europe. Peripheral CCCs are usually only noticeable above a certain size due to pain, fever, general sick feeling whilst the hilar or extrahepatic tumours are noticed earlier through the symptoms of obstructive jaundice. All in all, the prognosis of

CCC is unfavourable: infestation of neighbouring organs, lymphogenic metastasis and peritoneal carcinosis are frequently present at diagnosis. The hilar or extrahepatic tumours seem to have a rather better prognosis as they show up earlier through obstructive jaundice[24–26].

In tomographic diagnosis, reliable information on intra- and extrahepatic tumour spread must be obtained, taking the following points into consideration. In the case of cholangiocellular carcinoma, one usually finds irregular hypovascular space requirement with edge enhancement which can resemble colorectal metastases. In the case of the diffuse infiltrating type, detection of the tumour itself can be a problem. Focal atrophy, with cicatricial inclusions of the liver surface and increased serpentine expanded bile ducts due to tumour-induced fibrosis, are indeed characteristic but are very rare.

The central bile duct carcinoma (Klatskin tumour) remains a challenge for imaging procedures. MRCP (magnetic resonance cholangio-pancreatico-resonance tomography) is gaining increasing acceptance that is as an invasive procedure compared with ERCP[27–28]. Even after biliodigestive anastomosis, in which ERCP is not possible, MRCP is of great diagnostic assistance.

METASTASES

In cases with well-known tumour symptoms the assignment of liver metastases is usually not difficult but lesion detection can cause difficulties. Here, it is possible, by steadily reducing the layer thickness in CT and by introducing liver-specific contrast agents, to markedly increase the detection rate of lesions. Depending on the primary tumour, e.g. neuroendocrine tumour, the contrast agent dynamics and thus the biphasic spiral CT investigation of the liver play a large role. Tumour types, such as rhabdomyosarcoma, angiosarcoma and others, can rarely be differentiated. In principle, resection of liver metastases is indicated when an extrahepatic recidivous occurrence or a second tumour is excluded. It has been shown that a complete healthily resected metastasis (RO resection) and extrahepatic tumour infestation are the deciding prognostic factors[29,30]. Thus, in turn, the question of technical and functional resectability and questions of lymph node or distant metastases are of decisive importance.

As, in contrast to HCC, there is usually no cirrhosis in cases of liver metastases, resection is usually indicated. The 5-year survival rate after resection of colorectal liver metastases is 35–40%[31,32]. Recidivous resections had no significantly worse prognosis if it was possible to carry out an RO resection[33,34]. The 5-year survival rates for non-colorectal liver metastases are usually lower and are dependent on the primary tumour[35,36].

DIAGNOSTIC DIFFERENTIATION OF BENIGN LIVER TUMOUR

The use of modern imaging procedures has also increasingly revealed benign liver tumours. In everyday clinical practice, one frequently encounters haemangioma, liver cell adenoma or a focal–nodular hyperplasia.

The cavernous haemangioma is the most common benign liver tumour with a prevalence of 5–7% and a clearly more frequent occurrence in women. These inborn changes are often located subcapsularly and have the appearance of small dark-blue soft discrete tumours. The haemangiomas usually become symptomatic only above a certain size with non-specific stomach complaints. Sonographically, they show a homogenous echo-rich sharply delineated lesion. In over 20%, atypical haemangiomas with mixed echo patterns occur, usually in large haemangiomas with fibrotic and thrombotic portions which have to be further clarified diagnostically. Liver haemangiomas can today be reliably diagnosed on the basis of their typical contrast agent behaviour, the so-called iris shutter phenomenon in CT and MRT. Over all, rupture and the risk of bleeding are very small. Only in rare cases of haemangiomas is there an indication for operation after exclusion of other causes, for particular complaints or in cases with rapid increase in size ('giant haemangiomas'). The haemangiomas are scraped out. Arterial embolization does not appear to be indicated, owing to the risk of necrosis and its complications.

Hepatic adenoma occurs less frequently than haemangioma. This is a benign tumour made up of hepatocytes with uniform vascular architecture and missing bile ducts. Its appearance is a soft bright-yellow tumour, usually sharply delineated from the surrounding liver tissue. There is a high indication of a link with the intake of hormonal contraceptives and with glycogen storage disease type Ia. Sonographically, the tumour is, as a rule, discrete with an inhomogeneous echo pattern. In CT, the adenoma may also be discrete and, depending on the fat and blood perfusion portion, is hypo-, iso- or hyperdense. MRT investigation can help to further different diagnostic delineation. Unfortunately, the differential diagnosis between FNH, adenoma and highly differentiated HCC remains problematic even with modern diagnostics[37,38]. If doubts persist, even with medium-term ongoing check-ups, the hepatic adenoma is an indication for operation because of its malignant degeneration into hepatocellular carcinoma in up to 10% of cases.

Focal nodular hyperplasia has a prevalence of 2%; mostly, women are affected. Its relationship with the intake of hormonal contraceptives has not been clearly explained. Oestrogens promote its growth but do not appear to induce it. Focal nodular hyperplasias are tumour-like polycyclic nodal lesions with a central scar. Histologically, ductular proliferations around the fibre septa are typical.

Sonographically, in the case of FNH, a rather poorer echo pattern is usually found. Early lesions show an arterial homogeneous enhancement in CT and MRT, in which there is no central scar. In the late phase, the scar then shows a delayed enhancement. Imaging is over 75% conclusive. FNH is not an indication that an operation is required provided there is a clear reliable diagnosis: malignant transformations are not known.

SUMMARY

The operative treatment of liver tumours remains a great challenge. Advances of modern imaging have succeeded in achieving both early detection, on the one hand, and better characterization of the liver lesions, on the other. By this means, indications are clearer, operations better planned, and the number of unnecessary explorative laparotomies lowered. In cases with special problems, postprocessing procedures for volumetrization can be used. Of the many diagnostic possibilities, ultrasonic technology is a simple low-cost screening method for beginning the imaging procedure. Computer tomography and magnetic resonance tomography have the dominant role in further clarification as the best methods of detection. Other procedures, such as scintigraphy, positron emission tomography and angiography, are reserved for special indications. The diagnostic procedures should be timely, cost-effective and of low risk to the patient; they should have the highest possible specificity and sensitivity. The selection and sequence of diagnostic procedures is dependent on the clinical problem and requires close co-operation between surgeon and radiologist in order to avoid unnecessary multiple costly investigations.

References

1. Lehnert T, Otto G, Herfarth C. Therapeutic modalities and prognostic factors for primary and secondary liver tumors. World J Surg. 1995 Mar;19(2):252–63.
2. Scheele J, Stang R, Altendorf-Hofmann A, Paul M. Resection of colorectal liver metastases. World J Surg. 1995 Jan;19(1):59–71.
3. Harrison LE, Brennan MF, Newman E, Fortner JG, Picardo A, Blumgart LH, Fong Y. Hepatic resection for noncolorectal, nonneuroendocrine metastases: a fifteen-year experience with ninety-six patients. Surgery. 1997 Jun;121(6):625–32.
4. Schwartz SI. Hepatic resection for noncolorectal nonneuroendocrine metastases. World J Surg. 1995 Jan;19(1):72–5.
5. Seifert JK, Junginger T. Liver resections of metastases of non-colorectal primary tumors. Chirurg. 1996 Feb;67(2):161–8.
6. Pichlmayr R, Bretschneider HJ, Kirchner E, Ringe B, Lamesch P, Gubernatis G, Hauss J, Niehaus KJ, Kaukemuller J. [Ex situ operation on the liver. A new possibility in liver surgery]. Langenbecks Arch Chir. 1988;373(2):122–6.
7. Raab R, Schlitt HJ, Oldhafer KJ, Bornscheuer A, Lang H, Pichlmayr R. *Ex-vivo* resection techniques in tissue-preserving surgery for liver malignancies. Langenbecks Arch Surg. 2000 Apr;385(3):179–4.
8. Tsao JI, Lofhus JP, Nagorney DM, Adson MA, Ilstrup DM. Trends in morbidity and mortality of hepatic resection for malignancy: a matched comparative analysis. Ann Surg. 1994 220:199–205.
9. Oldhafer KJ, Hogemann D, Stamm G, Raab R, Peitgen HO, Galanski M. 3-dimensional (3-D) visualization of the liver for planning extensive liver resections. Chirurg. 1999 Mar;70(3):233–8.
10. Engstrom PF, Mc Glynn K, Hoffmann JP. Primary neoplasms of the liver. In: Holland JF, Bast RC Morton DL, Frei E, Kufe DW, Weichselbaum RR (eds) Canver medicine 4th edn. Williams and Wilkins, Balitmore. 1997, pp. 1923–38.
11. Khakoo SI, Grellier LF, Soni PN, Bhattacharya S, Dusheiko GM. Etiology, screening, and treatment of hepatocellular carcinoma. Med Clin North Am. 1996;80(5):1121–45.
12. Colombo M. Hepatocellular carcinoma. J Hepatol. 1992;15(1–2):225–36.
13. Belghiti J, Panis Y, Farges O, Benhamou JP, Fekete F. Intrahepatic recurrence after resection of hepatocellular carcinoma complicating cirrhosis. Ann Surg. 1991;214(2):114–17.
14. Iwatsuki S, Gordon RD, Shaw BJ, Starzl TE. Role of liver transplantation in cancer therapy. Annals of Surgery. 1985;202:401–7.
15. Yokoyama I, Todo S, Iwatsuki S, Starzl TE. Liver transplantation in the treatment of primary liver cancer Hepatogastroenterology. 1990;37 188–93.
16. Bismuth H, Chiche L, Adam R, Castaing D, Diamond T, Dennison A. Liver resection versus transplantation for hepatocellular carcinoma in cirrhotic patients. Ann Surg. 1993;218(2):145–51.
17. Romani F, Belli LS, Rondinara GF. The role of transplantation in small hepatocellular carcinoma complicating cirrhosis of the liver Journal of the American College of Surgeons. 1994; 178:379–84.
18. Mazzaferro V, Regalia E, Doci R, Andreola S, Pulvirenti A, Bozzetti F, Montalto F, Ammatuna M, Morabito A, Gennari L. Liver transplantation for the treatment of small hepatocellular carcinomas in patients with cirrhosis. N Engl J Med. 1996;334(11):693–9.

19. Michel J, Suc B, Montpeyroux F, Hachemanne S, Blanc P, Domergue J, Mouiel J, Gouillat C, Ducerf C, Saric J, Le Treut YP, Fourtanier G, Escat J. Liver resection or transplantation for hepatocellular carcinoma? Retrospective analysis of 215 patients with cirrhosis. J Hepatol. 1997; 26(6):1274-80.
20. Pinna AD, Iwatsuki S, Lee RG, Todo S, adariaga JR, Marsh JW, Casavilla A, Dvorchik I, Fung JJ, Starzl TE. Treatment of fibrlamellar hepatoma with subtotal hepatectomy or transplantation. Hepatology. 1997;26:877-83.
21. Pilchmayr R, Weimann A, Oldhafer KJ. Appraisal of transplantation for malignant tumours of the liver with special reference to early stage hepatocellular carcinoma. European Journal of Surgical Oncology. 1998;24:60-7.
22. Klintmalm GB. Liver transplantation for hepatocellular carcinoma – a registry report of the impact of tumor characteristics on outcome. Ann Surg. 1998;228:479-90.
23. Jonas S, Bechstein WO, Steinmuller T, Herrmann M, Radke C, Berg T, Settmacher U, Neuhaus P. Vascular invasion and histopathologic grading determine outcome after liver transplantation for hepatocellular carcinoma in cirrhosis. Hepatology. 2001;33(5):1080-6.
24. Pichlmayr R, Lamesch P, Weimann A, Tusch G, Ringe B. Surgical treatment of cholangiocellular carcinoma. World J Surg. 1995 Jan;19(1):83-8.
25. Klempnauer J, Ridder GJ, Werner M, Weimann A, Pichlmayr R. What constitutes long-term survival after surgery for hilar cholangiocarcinoma? Cancer. 1997 Jan 1;79(1):26-34.
26. Weimann A, Varnholt H, Schlitt HJ, Lang H, Flemming P, Hustedt C, Tusch G, Raab R. Retrospective analysis of prognostic factors after liver resection and transplantation for cholangiocellular carcinoma. Br J Surg. 2000 Sep;87(9):1182-7.
27. Hintze RE, Abou-Rebyeh H, Adler A, Veltzke-Schlieker W, Felix R, Wiedenmann B. Magnetic resonance cholangiopancreatography-guided unilateral endoscopic stent placement for Klatskin tumors. Gastrointest Endosc. 2001 Jan;53(1):40-6.
28. Yeh TS, Jan YY, Tseng JH, Chiu CT, Chen TC, Hwang TL, Chen MF. Malignant perihilar biliary obstruction: magnetic resonance cholangiopancreatographic findings. Am J Gastroenterol. 2000 Feb;95(2):432-40.
29. Beckurts KT, Holscher AH, Thorban S, Bollschweiler E, Siewert JR. Significance of lymph node involvement at the hepatic hilum in the resection of colorectal liver metastases. Br J Surg. 1997 Aug;84(8):1081-4.
30. Rodgers MS, McCall JL. Surgery for colorectal liver metastases with hepatic lymph node involvement: a systematic review. Br J Surg. 2000 Sep;87(9):1142-55.
31. Fong Y. Surgical therapy of hepatic colorectal metastasis. CA Cancer J Clin. 1999 Jul-Aug; 49(4):231-55.
32. Rees M, Plant G, Bygrave S. Late results justify resection for multiple hepatic metastases from colorectal cancer. Br J Surg. 1997 Aug;84(8):1136-40.
33. Herfarth C, Heuschen UA, Lamade W, Lehnert T, Otto G. Resections of recurrence in the liver of primary and secondary liver cancers. Chirurg. 1995 Oct;66(10):949-58.
34. Adam R, Bismuth H, Castaing D, Waechter F, Navarro F, Abascal A, Majno P, Engerran L. Repeat hepatectomy for colorectal liver metastases. Ann Surg. 1997 Jan;225(1):51-60.
35. Klempnauer J, Ridder GJ, Piso P, Pichlmayr R. Is liver resection in metastases of exocrine pancreatic carcinoma justified? Chirurg. 1996 Apr;67(4):366-70.
36. Lang H, Nussbaum KT, Weimann A, Raab R. Liver resection for non-colorectal, non-neuroendocrine hepatic metastases. Chirurg. 1999 Apr;70(4):439-46.
37. Flemming P, Wilkens L, Kreipe HH. Histopathological diagnosis of primary liver tumors. Pathologe. 2001 May;22(3):184-90.
38. Delorme S. Radiological diagnosis of the liver. Radiologe. 2000 Oct;40(10):904-15.

Section IV
Co-existence of imaging techniques

9
Scintigraphy/positron emission tomography (PET) – complementary support for endoscopy

W. H. KNAPP, K. F. GRATZ and A. R. BÖRNER

INTRODUCTION

Diagnostic nuclear medicine procedures complementary to endoscopy comprise a number of different imaging techniques such as static and dynamic conventional scintigraphy, single-photon emission tomography (SPET) as well as positron emission tomography (PET), and the use of different radiopharmaceuticals. The armamentarium of nuclear imaging methods is targeted to the following problems:

1. gastro-intestinal bleeding
2. oesophageal dysfunction
3. hepatic space-occupying lesions
4. detection of carcinomas with PET
5. endocrine tumours.

GASTROINTESTINAL BLEEDING

Methods

Extracorporeal labelling of red blood cells with Tc-99m and intravenous reinjection of 400–800 MBq is the preferred technique to radiolabel the intravascular space for periods as long as required until extravasation of red cells occurs. Immediately post-injection continuous imaging of the abdomen every 3 s is recommended. Since the initial images show only the large vessels, they help to localize exactly a source of bleeding in the acute stages. If there is no acute bleeding, static images of the whole abdomen, including the adjacent part of the thorax, should be recorded in anterior view. This imaging is recommended to be repeated every 1–2 h until the source of bleeding is localized. Often images taken as late as 24 h post-administration of the radiopharmaceutical are required.

Results

Extravasate into the intestinal lumen is characterized by a focal area with increasing count density in subsequent images and/or by focal activity accumulation showing dislocation according to the topography of the intestines. Thus, the small intestine can be differentiated from the colon by the pattern of activity displacement. Highly vascularized lesions can be detected by an intense focal count density during the early phase after administration of the activity (dynamic imaging). Sensitivity for detection of extravasation >0.05–0.1 ml/min exceeds 90% (acute or repetitive bleeding).

Problems

The intravascular space may be superposed by activity in the urinary tract and/or in the kidneys, in particular, if the labelling yield of cells is compromised. Localization is achievable only when there is acute bleeding within 24 h post initiation of study.

Indications

1. Localization of leakage site.
2. Immediately after emergency hospitalization due to intestinal bleeding (actual bleeding is needed to correctly localize source).

OESOPHAGEAL DYSFUNCTION

Oesophageal functional scintigraphy is supplementary to morphological X-ray imaging with barium contrast media and to endoscopy in physiological and quantitative assessment of oesophageal transport and function of the cardia. By this quantitative imaging approach, oesophageal dysfunction and gastro-oesophageal reflux can be detected.

Methods

First, 40 MBq Tc-99m sulphur colloid or DTPA are mixed with liquid or solid test meals. Immediately after oral administration and a single swallow rapid sequences of imaging (2 s intervals) is begun for a period of 2 min. During a further (subsequent) period of 10 min images are acquired for 30 s each. Evaluation is based on the 'region-of-interest' technique which allows one to display time–activity curves of different segments of the oesophagus (proximal, medial and distal thirds). The following parameters can be obtained: percentage void after 10–15 s, mean transit time, etc. The analysis of data in a single comprehensive functional image (condensed image) allows presentation of the whole action of meal transport with temporal and spatial information within one image.

In order to detect and quantify gastro-oesophageal reflux, imaging is begun when activity has been completely eliminated from the oesophagus together with the onset of increasing abdominal pressure. Again, the 'region-of-interest' technique is used to calculate the relationship between ascending oesophageal activity and activity remaining in the stomach.

Results

The normal time of passage is >15 s, and about 10% of activity remains in the distal third of the oesophagus under physiological conditions. In case of oesophageal strictures or of aganglionary achalasia there is significantly reduced peristaltic displacement in the lower oesophageal segments, so that most commonly >50% of administered activity remains in the lower two-thirds of the oesophagus even after several actions of swallowing. If manometry is used as reference method for differentiating normal and pathological conditions, the sensitivity of functional scintigraphy using liquid test meals is 85% at a specificity of 90%.

In evaluating for gastro-oesophageal reflux, ratios of oesophageal/gastric activities <5% are regarded as normal. In children (<2 years) reflux of greater amounts is common, and does not indicate pathological conditions if this occurs only in the distal one-third of the oesophagus. The accuracy of the method is about 85%, and it is thus superior to endoscopy and radiological methods. Only long-term pH measurements are more accurate.

Indications

Diagnostic and quantitative assessment of primary and secondary impairment of oesophageal motility. In children who do not tolerate manometry well, oesophageal scintigraphy is the method of choice for assessing oesophageal dysfunction and gastro-oesophageal reflux.

HEPATIC SPACE-OCCUPYING LESIONS

The widespread use of sensitive methods of hepatic imaging, in particular sonography, allows us to detect a large number of intrahepatic lesions, of which the great majority have a good prognosis and need no intervention. In order to verify benignity the diagnostic test needs high specificity. Nuclear medicine provides pathophysiological information highly specific for the major benign hepatic lesions.

Methods

Blood pool imaging

Labelling of red blood cells *ex vivo* and reinjection of radioagent. Rapid sequential imaging post-injection for flow imaging, and late imaging (2 h post-injection) of intravascular volume. For lesions <3 cm single-photon emission tomography (SPET) is mandatory.

Hepatobiliary scintigraphy

Tc-99m labelled imino-diacetic-acetate derivatives (IDA), intravenous administration of 300–400 MBq with subsequent rapid imaging for about 1 min, followed by sequential imaging at 5-min intervals until 60 min post-injection. Early images show blood flow in large vessels, sequential imaging until about 10 min post-injection (four views), transport of radiopharmaceutical by hepatocytes (parenchyma phase), and delayed images (<50 min) show biliary tract and elimination of bile into gut.

Results

The sensitivity of blood pool scintigraphy for detection of haemangiomas depends largely on tumour size: it approximates 100% in tumours >2 cm, 80% in tumours 1–2 cm, and is below 50% in tumours <1.4 cm. With recent three-dimensional dynamic display techniques sensitivity may be further increased, so that even for lesions of 1 cm a sensitivity of about 80% appears realistic. Haemangiomas are characterized by an increased blood pool in combination with decreased blood flow. The exchange of the blood pool progresses from the circumference in centripedal direction (or vice-versa). Only in a small percentage (<10%) there may be arterial delivery with rapid blood exchange. Correspondingly, the typical patterns in blood pool imaging are early count deficiency and delayed positive contrast in the area of the lesion. If these typical criteria are fulfilled the specificity of the method approximates 100%. Lack of early count deficiency logically (see above) does not exclude haemangioma; however, without this sign specificity of increased blood pool as shown by scintigraphy in the delayed phase is only 85–95%. In our patient population ($n = 530$), we found positive delayed contrast (of moderate intensity) for lesions other than haemangiomas in one case of focal nodular hyperplasia (FNH), in one case of adenoma, in one metastasis of colon carcinoma and in one patient with hepatic arteriovenous malformation. This extremely low incidence in our own observations is in agreement with the data reported in the literature. Only a few false-positive results have been described, e.g., caused by haemangiosarcoma and by hepatocellular carcinoma (HCE).

In focal nodular hyperplasia (FNH) there is typically increased perfusion and normal or increased density of hepatocytes in combination with dysfunction of small biliary ducts. Therefore, there are three typical decisive criteria necessary for verifying FNH by hepatobiliar scintigraphy:

1. positive contrast in initial images (in-flow phase of activity);
2. normal count density or positive contrast during the parenchyma phase;
3. positive contrast in the delayed phase (when activity has disappeared from normal liver).

If all three criteria are fulfilled the specificity approximates 100%. The sensitivity ranges between 86% and 90%. In our own patient population only one result out of those of 169 patients showing the above three criteria proved false-positive. Sensitivity and specificity of magnetic resonance imaging are – for comparison – about 70–98%. It is important to mention that late activity trapping does not suffice for diagnosis of FNH, as HCC show positive contrast in the delayed phase in 37%, and 66% of this subgroup show, in addition, hypervascularization (positive contrast in the in-flow phase). Therefore, the parenchyma phase has an essential role for differentiation, as 87% of HCC show negative contrasts.

Problems

Whereas positive contrasts are produced by even very small tumours, count deficiencies are obtained only when lesions exceed a volume of 1–2 cm. Since count deficiency may be important for specificity in haemangioma imaging, or for differential diagnosis between FNH and HCC, diagnostic accuracy is compromised in small lesions, in particular when located in dorsal areas where superposition with aorta or kidney may complicate reading of planar images. In images non-diagnostic as to vascularity of lesions, interpretation of scintigraphy should be combined with results of coloured Doppler sonography or angiography.

Indications

Space-occupying lesions detected with sonography, if there is a high probability of benignity, in particular in hypervascularized tumours, if greater than 1–2 cm.

DETECTION OF CARCINOMAS WITH PET

PET with (F-18)fluorodeoxyglucose (FDG) is nowadays recognized as an important tool in oncology, and its role for staging, detection of recurrences and therapy monitoring has been defined for a number of tumour entities. In gastroenterology FDG PET is employed for gastro-oesophageal, hepatocellular, pancreatic and colorectal cancer, the latter of which has the greatest relevance.

Methods

Gastrointestinal carcinoma cells show significant overexpression of glucose transporter and glycolytic key enzymes. FDG undergoes intracellular transport and phosphorylation in analogy to glucose. FDG-6-phosphate, however, is not further metabolized and is released from the cells only in very small amounts. Therefore, activity is trapped in cells with high glucose utilization. Fluorine-18 is produced with a cyclotron and has a half-life of 110 min. Therefore, synthesis of FDG, quality control, delivery to the application site and administration to the patient require perfect organization.

The radiopharmaceutical has to be injected after at least 5 h; better after overnight fasting of the patient. Glucose serum levels should not exceed 6 mmol/L. Therefore, actual glucose levels should be determined immediately prior to the onset of the investigation. If necessary, normalization of glucose level has to be obtained before administration of FDG. In some individuals, medication for muscle relaxation (butyl scopolamine) may be required to avoid significant FDG uptake in musculature. PET imaging (several bed positions so that the body from neck to pelvis is included) is begun 45–60 min post-injection. In rectal carcinoma the bladder must be voided before the onset of imaging, and catheterization is recommended. There are various modalities to display the three-dimensional information on intracorporeal activity distribution: maximum intensity projections (MIPS) for an overview to detect lesions of unknown location, contiguous slices in three orientations (transversal, sagittal, coronal) for suspected locations, and multi-modality imaging using fusion software for magnetic resonance imaging (MRI) and computerized tomography (CT).

Results

Gastro-oesophageal cancer

The key patient management issues for using FDG PET are staging for possible spread of tumour and assessing recurrence. In terms of sensitivity the accuracy in primary tumour detection is superior to that of detection of lymph node metastases (94–100% versus 45–76%). Lymph node staging, however, is clinically more important, as CT scans can show lymph node enlargement when no tumour is present. On the other hand, lymph node metastases as shown in PET scans may not be enlarged. Therefore, sensitivity of CT in detection of lymph node metastases is reported to be only 29–75%, and specificity in initial staging as low as 29%, whereas the specificity of positive PET scans is 90%[1–3]. Similar differences in accuracy between PET and CT have been observed in staging of distant metastases: sensitivity and specificity of PET 69–100% and 93% versus the corresponding values for CT, 46% and 74%. Therefore, including PET in patient management was found to cause a 20% change of treatment (meta-analysis of 229 patient studies)[4]. In the diagnosis of recurrence PET approximates a sensitivity of 100%; the overall specificity, however, was reported as 43% (see 'Problems')[4].

Hepatocellular cancer

Since hepatocellular carcinoma is associated with cirrhosis in 50–80% of patients, and since 5% of patients with cirrhosis eventually develop hepatocellular cancer, the key management issue for FDG PET is distinguishing between cirrhosis and hepatoma. As surgery is the treatment of choice only for patients with localized disease, a second issue is identifying or excluding multifocal lesions. Finally, FDG PET can be used for assessing response to treatment and differentiating tumour from necrosis, oedema, and scarring. Reliable data (patient populations with $n > 100$) from the literature are actually available only for the accuracy in staging: sensitivity and specificity for PET 77% and 97% versus CT 38% and 97%[4,5].

Pancreatic cancer

Considering the poor prognosis in patients with pancreatic carcinomas, FDG PET may perform a clinical role in helping to characterize lesions appearing in the pancreas. The key issues for employment of FDG PET are differentiating chronic pancreatic masses from cancer, staging nodal and liver metastases, and assessing response to chemotherapy. The sensitivity of PET in primary diagnosis is reported at 90–96% with specificities of 82–100%[6–8]. The corresponding values for CT are 69–89% and 69–100%. The accuracy of FDG PET in staging depends largely (like that of CT) on the size of lymph node involvement. The overall sensitivity was reported as 68%; in metastases >1 cm, however, 97%, and in metastases <1 cm 43%[5]. The data for specificity range between 84% and

95%. Quantitation of PET scans by using 'standardized uptake values' (SUV) does not increase overall accuracy, but allows us to better define with which degree of sensitivity or specificity scans are to be read. For example, to obtain a 100% specificity in detecting malignancies with PET, a cut-off of SUV = 3 is to be applied. A cut-off level as high as this, however, decreases sensitivity to 87–88%[4]. The data actually available for monitoring response do not yet allow statistically valid interpretation and comparison with other imaging modalities. In two studies including a total of 31 patients a sensitivity of monitoring response was 92% at a specificity of 100%[9,10].

Colorectal cancer

Diagnostics in colorectal cancer is the most important application of FDG PET in gastroenterology. Primary treatment is surgical, but >50% of patients have recurring cancers, of which about 20% are eligible for further surgical resection. Every second patient has relapsing cancer because of previously unidentified metastases. After determination of tumour spread (localization and definition of number of metastases) it can be decided whether surgery for removal of metastases (e.g. of the liver) may be an option. Therefore, key issues for PET imaging are evaluating suspected recurrence and restaging, assessing response to treatment, and evaluating liver lesions for metastatic disease (Figure 1).

There is nowadays a large body of evidence (studies in >1300 patients) that sensitivity and specificity of PET in detection of recurrence are superior to those of other modalities: PET 94% and 87% versus CT 79% and 73% on average[4]. The accuracy of both PET and CT in lymph node staging is unsatisfactory as

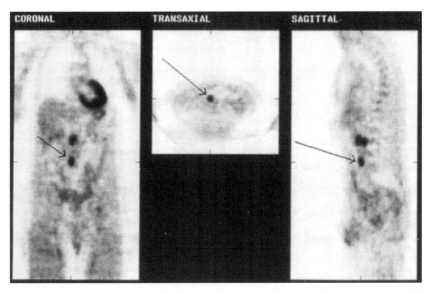

Figure 1 Six months post-surgery of colorectal carcinoma. Increase in CEA level. PET with FDG shows two abdominal metastases. The inferior (para-aortic) metastasis is shown on all 3 slices (arrows)

neither modality is sensitive enough (about 30%). An important advantage, however, of FDG PET is the high accuracy in detection of liver metastases with a sensitivity of near 90% and a specificity approximating 100%, whereas the sensitivity of CT is near 40% at the same specificity as PET[11–14]. The impact of FDG PET for patient management by staging and detection of recurrence exceeds 30% according to a meta-analysis of 236 and 915 patients, respectively[4].

Regarding the accuracy in monitoring response, again the number of data available in the literature is insufficient to draw valid statistical conclusions. In 30 patients, however, sensitivity and specificity range from 90% to 100%[15,16]. These values were obtained after 4–5 weeks of chemotherapy, with a ≥75% decrease in FDG uptake as criterion for response.

Problems

Post-radiotherapy, inflammatory reactions in the area of recurrence, as well as inflammatory lymph nodes, may cause increased FDG uptake and make the image indistinguishable from residual disease or lymph node metastases. Therefore, monitoring of radiotherapy response with FDG PET is of only limited value during a period of 6 months. The low sensitivity in detection of abdominal lymph node metastases is due to the heterogeneous FDG distribution pattern in the intestines.

Indications

Differential diagnoses, staging of lymph nodes and distant metastases, detection of recurrence, monitoring of therapy response. Indications of FDG PET for individual tumour entities, see above.

NEUROENDOCRINE TUMOURS

Since the introduction of radiolabelled somatostatin analogues nuclear medicine imaging has become useful to localize and stage tumours of the gastroenteropancreatic system with endocrine activity.

Methods

The first compound used for external imaging was octreotide labelled with I-123. Due to rapid deiodination this compound proved unsatisfactory. Instead, pentreotide with DTPA as linker for In-111 was introduced in clinical application, and the resulting radioligand is to date the only commercially available radiopharmaceutical for specific imaging of neuroendocrine tumours. About 200 MBq of this agent is injected intravenously without particular preceding preparation of patients. Even ongoing therapies with somatostatin analogues for therapy need not be discontinued. Whole-body imaging in anterior and posterior views is recommended 4 and 24 h post-injection, supplemented by emission tomography (SPET) 24 h and occasionally also 48 h post-injection. The 48 h imaging is in particular recommended when 24 h images show indeterminate abdominal findings. In order to avoid false-positive interpretations due to intestinal activity, laxantia should be given prior to late imaging. Recently a number of new radioligands have been synthesized and have undergone clinical testing. Of particular interest is a recent positron-emitting agent (Ga-68-DOTATOC), a radiopeptide linked to the chelator DOTA. This compound is rapidly eliminated from tissue where not specifically bound, so that there is almost no abdominal background activity. PET can be begun as early as 60 min post-injection[17]. This radioagent is, however, not yet commercially available.

Results

Somatostatin receptor imaging proved to be particularly useful in various tumours of the gastroenteropancreatic system with endocrine activity. Though it is relatively easy to establish the diagnosis of these tumours, due to their typical clinical symptoms and changes in serum parameters, it is often difficult to localize them. Somatostatin receptor scintigraphy allows us to identify >90% of tumour locations except in the case of insulinomas, in which the sensitivity is only about 50%. Sensitivity is limited in lesions <1 cm with conventional imaging (planar and SPET), smaller lesions may be better identified with recent (experimental) positron-emitting radioligands and PET (Figure 2).

Problems

Small tumours may not be identified (see above), uptake in liver, kidneys and gut may obscure tumour contrasts when using the commercial radiopharmaceutical. Sequential imaging can reduce, but not completely solve, this problem.

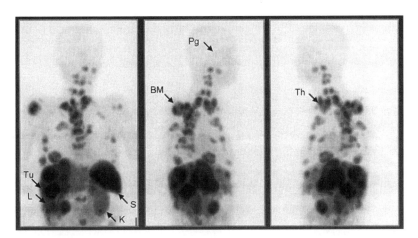

Figure 2 Multi-metastatic lesions of carcinoid. PET with Ga-68 DOTATOC shows lesions with high positive contrast 60 min post-injection. Even very small lesions are identified
BM = bone metastasis
K = kidney
L = liver
Pg = pineal gland
Th = thyroid
S = spleen
Tu = intrahepatic tumour location

Indications

Somatostatin receptor scintigraphy is indicated as a complementary imaging method in the diagnostics of localization and spread of carcinoids and other tumours of the gastroenteropancreatic system. It is particularly useful when surgical therapy is planned. In the realm of surgical interventions probe-based localization is an additional option. Scintigraphy may also be helpful in testing whether identified tumours express somatostatin receptors before therapy with somatostatin analogues is initiated. Therapy with radioactive somatostatin analogues (beta-rays and Auger electron-emitting radionuclides such as In-111, Y-90, and Ga-67) are under investigation. When this internal radiotherapy becomes more widely used, scintigraphy will be mandatory for treatment decisions and pretreatment dosimetry.

Perspective

In recent years several molecular targets have been identified as specific for individual tumour types. Progress in antibody technology and radiolabelling of constructs such as mini-antibodies or peptides may provide a greater number of efficient and highly specific imaging methods for various kinds of tumours. These developments may, in addition, open new avenues for treatment with radionuclides in minimal residual or disseminated disease.

References

1. Block M, Patterson G, Sundaresan R et al. Improvement in staging of esophageal cancer with addition of positron emission tomography. Ann Thorac Surg. 1997;64:770–6.
2. Meltzer CC, Luketich JD, Friedmann D et al. Whole-body FDG positron emission tomographic imaging for staging esophageal cancer. Comparison with computed tomography. Clin Nucl Med. 2000;25:882–7.
3. Luketich JD, Schauer PR, Meltzer CC et al. Role of positron emission tomography in staging esophageal cancer. Ann Thorac Surg. 1997;64:765–9.
4. Gambhir SS, Czernin J, Schwimmer J, Silverman DHS, Coleman RE, Phelps M. A tabulated summary of the FDG PET literature. J Nucl Med. 2001;42:1–93S.
5. Fröhlich A, Diederichs C, Staib L, Vogel J, Beger H, Reske S. Detection of liver metastases from pancreatic cancer using FDG PET. J Nucl Med. 1999;40:250–5.
6. Friess H, Langhans J, Ebert M et al. Diagnosis of pancreatic cancer by 2(18F)-fluoro-2-deoxy-D-glucose positron emission tomography. Gut. 1995;36:771–7.
7. Stollfuss JC, Glatting G, Friess H, Kocher F, Berger HG, Reske SN. 2-(Fluorine-18)-fluoro-2-deoxy-D-glucose PET in detection of pancreatic cancer: value of quantitative image interpretation. Radiology. 1995;195:339–44.
8. Imdahl A, Nitzsche E, Krautmann F et al. Evaluation of positron emission tomography with 2-(18F) fluoro-2-deoxy-D-glucose for the differentiation of chronic pancreatitis and pancreatic cancer. Br J Surg. 1999;86:194–9.
9. Shields AF, Ahmed S, Zalupski MM et al. FDG-PET evaluation of pancreatic cancer treatment. J Nucl Med. 1999;40:243P (abstract).
10. Higashi T, Sakahara H, Torizuka T et al. Evaluation of intraoperative radiation therapy for unresectable pancreatic cancer with FDG PET. J Nucl Med. 1999;40:1424–33.
11. Abdel-Nabi H, Dierr RJ, Lamonica DM et al. Staging of primary colorectal carcinomas with fluorine-18 fluorodeoxyglucose whole-body PET: correlation with histopathologic and CT findings. Radiology. 1998;206:755–60.
12. Whiteford MH, Whiteford HM, Yee LF et al. Usefulness of FDG-PET scan in the assessment of suspected metastatic or recurrent adenocarcinoma of the colon and rectum. Dis Colon Rectum. 2000;43:759–70.

13. Valk PE, Abella-Columna E, Hasemann MK et al. Whole-body PET imaging with F-18 fluorodeoxyglucose in management of recurrent colorectal cancer. Arch Surg. 1999;134:503–13.
14. Vitola JV, Delbeke D, Sandler MP et al. Positron emission tomography to stage suspected metastatic colorectal carcinoma to the liver. Am J Surg. 1996;171:21–6.
15. Bender H, Bangard N, Metten N et al. Possible role of FDG-PET in the early prediction of therapy outcome in liver metastases of colorectal cancer. Hybridoma. 1999;18:87–91.
16. Findlay M, Young H, Cunningham D et al. Noninvasive monitoring of tumor metabolism using fluorodeoxyglucose and positron emission tomography in colorectal cancer liver metastases: correlation with tumor response to fluoro-uracil (see comments). J Clin Oncol. 1996;14:700–8.
17. Hofmann M, Maecke H, Börner AR et al. Biokinetics and imaging with the somatostatin receptor PET radioligand 68Ga-DOTATOC: preliminary data. Eur J Nucl Med. 2001 (In press).

10
Magnetic resonance imaging: a substitute for endoscopy?

H. E. ADAMEK, J. ALBERT, H. BREER and J. F. RIEMANN

INTRODUCTION

Magnetic resonance imaging (MRI) has been called the most important development in medical diagnosis since the discovery of the X-ray more than 100 years ago. It has early become one of the major diagnostic tools in neuroradiology and is now being applied to virtually every part of the body. With the development of fast imaging sequences and special surface coils, and the improvements in the quality of abdominal images, MRI has come a long way in a short time. The effectiveness of MRI has been expanded to a variety of gastrointestinal disorders. The gastroenterologist's attention is currently focused on biliopancreatic and bowel diseases.

PANCREATIC–BILIARY DISEASES

The ability of MRI to depict a dilated biliary tract was first demonstrated in 1986. Five years later, magnetic resonance cholangiopancreatography (MRCP) was described for the first time as a completely non-invasive application which enables visualization of the biliary and pancreatic ducts similar to those of endoscopic retrograde cholangiopancreatography (ERCP) without the need for contrast material[1]. Recent technical advances have led to notable improvements in this field with a good toleration by patients and a surprising clinical acceptance by gastroenterologists.

MRCP was found to be highly sensitive (90–100%) in the visualization of the normal common bile duct. Furthermore, bile duct dilation is constantly visible during MRCP[2]. In the diagnosis of choledocholithiasis, MRCP reaches a sensitivity between 80% and 100% when modern techniques with strong gradients are employed. The sensitivity of MRCP for the detection of choledocholithiasis is superior to that of percutaneous ultrasonography and computerized tomography (CT). There are limitations for routine MRCP use with standard equipment for diagnosing common bile duct stones[3], particularly for stones smaller than 6 mm. Another potential error is the misdiagnosis of a stone as another type of intraluminal filling defect, such as an intraductal tumour, blood clot, or gas bubble.

Congenital biliary abnormalities are well depicted by MRCP. Extra- and intrahepatic dilation is adequately revealed in patients with choledochal cysts[4]. In hepatolithiasis, and for the diagnosis of primary sclerosing cholangitis, MRCP also proved to be useful[5].

There is currently no consensus on the precise role of MRCP in the clinical assessment of patients with suspected bile duct obstruction. Although the presence and site of biliary strictures can be identified by percutaneous ultrasonography, the evaluation of the cause of such strictures may be more difficult and requires direct cholangiopancreatography. ERCP often shows only the ducts below the site of obstruction (double-duct sign); visualization of an obstructed part of the biliary tree is often not possible. In addition, opacification of undrained bile ducts places the patient at risk of cholangitis. MRCP can detect the presence of biliary obstruction and its level with a sensitivity of about 90% and a specificity that reaches almost 100%. Furthermore, it routinely identifies the dilated biliary tree upstream of an obstruction, allowing synchronous strictures to be identified[6]. Nevertheless, the cause of such strictures may be more difficult to determine on the basis of MRCP alone. The differential diagnostic considerations can be improved with the use of conventional cross-sectional MR images. The role of MRCP in patients with an obstruction at the level of the ampulla has not been adequately studied. ERCP obviously has several advantages over MRCP in this group of patients, since it permits direct visualization of the ampulla, biopsy of lesions or intraductal sonography.

Due to the small calibre, the evaluation of the normal pancreatic duct has long been a major technical challenge for MRCP. Visualization of the pancreatic duct can be improved if imaging is performed using advanced techiques and after the administration of secretin. The administration of secretin is now recommended when the pancreatic duct is not apparent on MRCP[7]. Secretin-enhanced MRCP can also permit visualization of possible communications of the pancreatic duct with pseudocysts in patients with advanced chronic pancreatitis. Some authors even prophesy that dynamic secretion-enhanced MRCP, with the acquisition of multiple pictures at short intervals after stimulation, will improve the understanding of the pathophysiology of pancreatitis. Should the dynamic evaluation of the bile ducts after choleretic stimulation also come to reality, the performance of an ERCP to measure sphincter pressures manometrically is likely to become obsolete.

So far, MRCP has seldom been used in the setting of acute pancreatitis. Recent reports[8], however, have reported similar results between contrast-enhanced CT and non-enhanced MRCP in diagnosing pancreatic necrosis and acute fluid collections. As techniques continue to improve, MRCP might become the main imaging modality for patients with acute pancreatitis. Presently, MRCP has been shown to be of clear value in the diagnosis of chronic pancreatitis[9]. In the diagnosis of pancreas divisum and cystic, mucin-producing tumours of the pancreas, MRCP has been reported to be equal or even superior to ERCP[10]. This is also true for ductal pancreatic carcinoma, where MRCP is as sensitive as ERCP.

Furthermore, it is feasible to presume that the use of MRCP may prevent inappropriate explorations of the pancreatic and common bile ducts in cases of suspected pancreatic carcinoma, where interventional endoscopic therapy is unlikely[11]. Undoubtedly, MRCP is the method of choice in all patients with technically failed ERCP examinations[12].

BOWEL DISEASES

Imaging of the total small bowel is mainly performed using X-ray barium techniques, since enteroscopy is able to examine only a small section. MRI possesses many characteristics that would make it an ideal imaging technique for the small bowel[13]. Unfortunately its application is still limited due to some technical and practical drawbacks. A range of both positive and negative contrast media have been investigated, but until recently a suitable contrast medium to delineate the bowel was lacking. Once these and some other technical problems have been solved, MR enteroscopy is likely to become the preferable method for evaluating the entire small bowel.

Colonoscopy is the method of choice for the diagnosis of colon diseases. Continuing advances in the capability of the hardware used in MRI have made high-resolution data volumes available. With the aid of sophisticated algorithms and high-resolution two-dimensional high-resolution images, three-dimensional images of the colon, simulating those obtained with conventional colonoscopy, can be reconstructed off-line[14]. This rapidly growing field of 'virtual colonoscopy' has gained multidisciplinary attention as a potential non-invasive test for colorectal polyps and cancer[15–17], with the hope of overcoming many disadvantages associated with conventional endoscopy, including its invasiveness, patient discomfort, and the potential for iatrogenic perforation. Although marked technological advances have been achieved, the challenges that lie ahead include standardization, implementation of these techniques in generalized settings, and patient acceptance[18]. Currently, MR colonography is available at only a handful of centres throughout the world. The current cost consists of the time required for a radiologist to perform the procedure and the cost for the contrast agent[19]. The need for a subsequent colonoscopy to evaluate many false-positive results (low specificity) and resect polyps must also be included. As long as these problems are not sufficiently addressed, virtual colonoscopy is far from being promoted as a tool for general screening purposes in suspected colon diseases. It might at best be recommended for the preoperative assessment of the tumour stage of rectal cancer[20], and for evaluating the entire colon before surgery in patients with distal occlusive cancers, which cannot be traversed endoscopically[21].

SUMMARY

Whether or not the survival of diagnostic endoscopy is under debate, MRI could mark a historic turning point in gastroenterology. Conceivably, MRCP and MRI, together with magnetic resonance angiography (MRA), may prove most cost-effective in current preoperative staging practices for bile duct and pancreatic cancer with greatest patient acceptance. Gastroenterologists should not fear

MRI: A SUBSTITUTE FOR ENDOSCOPY?

MRI as potential competition for endoscopy, but should consider MRI to be a revolutionary development in gastroenterology; one that should be included into diagnostic algorithms.

References

1. Wallner BK, Schumacher KA, Weidenmaier W et al. Dilated biliary tract: evaluation with MR cholangiography with a T2-weighted contrast enhanced fast sequence. Radiology. 1991;181:805–8.
2. Soto JA, Barish MA, Yucel EK et al. Magnetic resonance cholangiography: comparison with endoscopic retrograde cholangiopancreatography. Gastroenterology. 1996;110:589–97.
3. Zidi SH, Prat F, Le Guen O et al. Use of magnetic resonance cholangiography in the diagnosis of choledocholithiasis: prospective comparison with a reference imaging method. Gut. 1999;44:118–22.
4. Adamek HE, Albert J, Weitz M et al. A prospective evaluation of magnetic resonance cholangiopancreatography in patients with suspected bile duct obstruction. Gut. 1998;43:680–3.
5. Kubo S, Hamba H, Hirohashi K et al. Magnetic resonance cholangiography in hepatolithiasis. Am J Gastroenterol. 1997;92:629–31.
6. Hintze RE, Adler A, Veltzke W et al. Clinical significance of magnetic resonance cholangiopancreatography (MRCP) compared with ERCP. Endoscopy. 1997;29:182–7.
7. Matos C, Metens T, Devière J et al. Pancreatic duct: morphologic and functional evaluation with dynamic MR pancreatography after secretin stimulation. Radiology. 1997;203:435–41.
8. Lecesne R, Taourel P, Bret PM et al. Acute pancreatitis: interobserver agreement and correlation of CT and MR cholangiopancreatography with outcome. Radiology. 1999;211:727–35.
9. Sica GT, Braver J, Cooney MJ et al. Comparison of endoscopic retrograde cholangiopancreatography with MR cholangiopancreatography in patients with pancreatitis. Radiology. 1999;210:605–10.
10. Albert J, Schilling D, Breer H, Jungius KP, Riemann JF, Adamek HE. Mucinous cystadenomas and intraductal papillary mucinous tumors of the pancreas in magnetic resonance cholangiopancreatography. Endoscopy. 2000;32:472–6.
11. Adamek HE, Albert J, Breer H, Weitz M, Schilling D, Riemann JF. Pancreatic cancer detection with magnetic resonance cholangiopancreatography and endoscopic retrograde cholangiopancreatography: a prospective controlled study. Lancet. 2000;356:190–3.
12. Adamek HE, Weitz M, Breer H et al. Value of magnetic resonance cholangiopancreatography (MRCP) after unsuccessful ERCP. Endoscopy. 1997;29:741–4.
13. Hansmann HJ, Hess T, Hahmann M et al. MRI for chronic inflammatory bowel disease. Fortschr Röntgenstr. 2001;173:4–11.
14. Luboldt W, Bauerfeind P, Steiner P et al. Preliminary assessment of three-dimensional magnetic resonance imaging for various colonic disorders. Lancet. 1997;349:1288–91.
15. Hara AK, Johnson CD, Reed JE et al. Detection of colorectal polyps by computed tomographic colography: feasibility of a novel technique. Gastroenterology. 1996;110:284–90.
16. Fenlon HM, Nunes DP, Schroy PC et al. A comparison of virtual and conventional colonoscopy for the detection of colorectal polyps. N Engl J Med. 1999;341:1496–503.
17. Rex DK, Vining D, Kopecky KK. An initial experience with screening for colon polyps using spiral CT with and without CT colonography. Gastrointest Endosc. 1999;50:309–13.
18. Mc Farland EG, Brink JA. Helical CT colonography (virtual colonoscopy): the challenge that exists between advancing technology and generalizability. Am J Roentgenol. 1999;173:549–59.
19. Luboldt W, Frohlich JM, Schneider N et al. MR colonography: optimized enema composition. Radiology. 1999;212:265–9.
20. Brown G, Richards CJ, Newcombe RG et al. Rectal carcinoma: thin-section MR imaging for staging in 28 patients. Radiology. 1999;211:215–22.
21. Fenlon HM, McAneny DB, Nunes DP et al. Occlusive colon carcinoma: virtual colonoscopy in the preoperative evaluation of the proximal colon. Radiology. 1999;210:423–8.

11
Three-dimensional (3D) imaging: from sectional image to 3D model

M. A. BARISH

INTRODUCTION

The role of radiological imaging is to demonstrate the existence or absence of pathology in the human body. Communicating these findings is as important as their identification, with proper display, presentation and transmission (either as film or electronically) of the images being essential. Unfortunately, pathological conditions in the human body rarely exist purely in an orthogonal plane such as the axial slices typically acquired in computerized tomography (CT). Although well-trained radiologists have the ability to mentally reconstruct these axial slices into a three-dimensional (3D) image, it is a taxing and time-consuming means of interpreting or transmitting information. Subsequent interpreters must repeat the mental reprocessing of the data to develop a 3D understanding of the pathological condition. In addition, non-radiologist clinicians may not be able to perform such mental reprocessing, requiring the radiologist to spend vital time attempting to communicate complex relationships. The conversion of a series of sectional or 2D slices into 3D models has the potential to reduce the time needed to both analyse and communicate complicated anatomical relationships. This has been one of the prime driving forces behind image processing and 3D imaging. This chapter will review the reasons for pursuing 3D imaging and the techniques involved, and will also review one of the most recent advancements in gastrointestinal imaging to capitalize on 3D imaging; virtual colonoscopy.

THE CASE FOR 3D IMAGING

The use of 3D imaging by radiologists has been previously limited to major academic imaging departments and usually performed for research rather than clinical purposes. The reasons for this are multifactorial and consist of a series of barriers to the routine implementation of 3D imaging. The cost of performing 3D reconstructions was a significant barrier to the widespread use of this technology. Workstations were major capital expenses usually tied to the purchase of CT or magnetic resonance imaging (MRI) scanners. Due to the high cost of the technology, most radiology departments purchased only a single workstation for the department, which limited access. In addition the user interfaces were difficult to understand, requiring training of special personnel, typically technologists, which further increased cost. The recent advances in computer processing power, data storage, and software-rendering algorithms now make it possible to develop 3D imaging workstations on inexpensive, easy-to-use personal computer, platforms which has significantly reduced cost.

A second former barrier to the implementation of 3D imaging included limited access to quality image data acceptable for post-processing. The widespread installation of helical and multi-detector CT scanners, modern MRI scanners, and PACS systems allows for the acquisition and distribution of high-resolution, thin-slice data which are necessary for the production of diagnostic high-quality 3D reconstructions. In fact, the newer multi-detector CT scanners acquire such a large number of slices that conventional methods of image review become obsolete. Future PACS image review workstations with 3D capability for reviewing multi-detector CT is likely to become the norm.

As 3D imaging becomes more available, inexpensive and easier to use, one can expect that the generation of 3D images will become part of the routine workflow of image interpretation. The widespread installation of multi-detector CT scanners is likely to require the fusion of 2D and 3D workstations for all softcopy CT reading stations further increasing the use of 3D images.

TECHNIQUES

When a set of parallel planar images are 'stacked' together, they can be considered as forming a 3D volume of data that can undergo post-processing through a wide variety of techniques. The most common of these techniques are multi-planar reformat, maximum-intensity projection, surface-shaded rendering, and volume rendering. Each of these types of processing or rendering has unique advantages and disadvantages but several general principles apply. In all types of 3D post-processing the most important determinants of image quality relate to the relative sizes of the voxels and the amount of noise within the data. For optimum image quality the pixels should be as close to cubic as possible. This means that, in the case of CT imaging, the slice thickness should be as close as possible to the field of view divided by the pixel matrix size. For example, in a typical scan the field of view is approximately 40 cm, while the pixel matrix size is 512×512 pixels. This results in a pixel size of approximately 0.8 mm. If the slice thickness is 1 mm then the pixels will be nearly cubic. However, in most CT systems, as the slice thickness decreases, either the inherent image noise (quantum mottle) or the effective radiation dose to the patient will increase. This balance between image quality and radiation dose must be assessed for the specific study being performed.

Multi-planar reformation

One of the most frequently used techniques, and perhaps the simplest, is the technique of multi-planar reformation (MPR). Typically, CT images are acquired as a series of parallel axial slices that are perpendicular to the long axis of the body. However, often the radiologist or interpreting physician wishes to inspect the anatomy in an alternative plane to the plane of acquisition. This can be accomplished by the use of MPR, in which the set of axial slices are interpolated between the first and last slice to create a 3D volume. Interpolation is used to correct for the fact that the resolution within each slice (in-plane resolution) is typically in the range 0.5–1.0 mm while slice thickness is typically 2.5–10 mm. The slices are interpolated to obtain near-cubic voxels and reduce artifacts, such as the stair-step artifact. Stair-step artifact is also reduced when using multi-detector as compared to single-detector CT systems[1]. The derived image planes can be in any direction (such as sagittal, coronal or oblique) and in fact can even be described as complex curves. The uses of MPR images in gastrointestinal (GI) radiology are numerous and continue to increase with the introduction of multi-detector CT. For example, Wong et al.[2] reported the use of sagittal and coronal reformats in the evaluation of liver metastases and found that 'reformations provided a unique perspective with which to view the liver and may improve diagnostic capacity'. Curved MPRs have been used to evaluate vascular structures[3] and can also be used to 'straighten' the colon for use in virtual colonoscopy.

Maximum-intensity projection (MIP)

In this method of image post-processing the brightest pixel along a line is projected on to a 2D image. The direction of the line can be varied so as to create a series of images from all directions. In the case of CT data the pixels in the resultant 2D image contain only the Hounsfield unit value of the brightest voxel within the volume along the ray or line. The process loses all other data. The algorithm can be varied to choose either the minimum-intensity pixel or to sum (or average) all the pixel values along the line or ray. Unlike the MPR technique the resultant image contains data from portions throughout the 3D volume. Although this is a 3D processing technique, the projected image lacks a sense of depth or 3D quality since, to the viewer, one cannot ascertain from the final image where in the volume the resultant pixels were located. This can be slightly reduced by obtaining MIP images from multiple directions and viewing them in rapid succession to simulate a 'movie loop' or cine. MIP images have been used extensively in vascular imaging and a complete review of the literature is beyond the scope of this chapter.

Surface rendering

Surface rendering is based on the concept of thresholding, in which one chooses a value below which voxels are deemed unimportant. Once this threshold is set, each individual voxel is classified as belonging to one of two classes: visible voxels or non-visible voxels. A ray or line is then cast into the volume and the first visible voxel traversed is projected into the final image. All voxels behind this first voxel do not contribute to the final image. This technique is simple to use and able to be performed on inexpensive computer platforms. The addition of lighting, reflection, and shadows adds depth cues that create a realistic 3D image. However, only the surface of the structure can be displayed, limiting the reality effect. Difficulties also exist since the threshold needed to display certain anatomy can vary due to variations between patients, contrast enhancement, pathology and technique. In addition, surface rendering is very susceptible to image noise. Surface rendering has been used to display vascular anatomy, liver surface architecture, and for virtual colonoscopy[4].

Volume rendering

Volume rendering has many advantages over other 3D imaging techniques. Unlike MPR and MIP techniques, volume rendering has the advantage of depth cues and, unlike surface rendering, volume rendering has the ability to render the internal structure of objects. The idea behind volume rendering is to create a 2D image that represents the full structure of a 3D object. In volume rendering using CT data, rays are cast into the volume and take account of the Hounsfield unit values of each voxel within the volume. Each voxel along the ray is assigned an opacity value between 0% and 100%. The opacity value is determined from the brightness of the voxel (Hounsfield unit number or signal intensity) based on an opacity function. This function is usually a ramp or series of ramps along the intensity histogram. Each voxel is also considered to transmit, emit and reflect light. If a voxel is completely opaque (100%) then it will not transmit any light and will completely obscure objects behind the voxel. The resultant projection image is based on a compilation of the emitted, transmitted and reflected light along this ray. Therefore, the contribution that each voxel makes to the resultant image is based on the voxel's position and the voxel's Hounsfield unit (CT data) value or signal intensity (MRI data). It should be noted that shaded surface rendering could be thought of as a specific case of volume rendering where the opacity function is a step-function instead of a ramp and the opacity of all voxels above the threshold is set to 100%. A complete review of the detailed mathematical functions, artifacts, advantages and disadvantages of volume rendering is beyond the scope of this chapter. For an excellent review of this subject-matter one should read the review by Calhoun et al.[5]. Volume rendering has been used in a wide variety of GI imaging applications from liver anatomy[6], vascular anatomy[3,7], biliary anatomy[8], to virtual endoscopy[4]. It is this last application that has now placed the GI radiologist back into the arena of colorectal cancer screening, and will be the subject of the remainder of this chapter.

VIRTUAL COLONOSCOPY

Virtual colonoscopy or CT colonography is a promising new method for colorectal cancer screening. Helical computerized tomography (CT) is used to generate high-resolution, 2D axial images of the abdomen and pelvis. Three-dimensional images of the colon simulating those obtained with conventional colonoscopy can be reconstructed from the data obtained, using either surface rendering or volume rendering as previously described[4]. Favourable attributes of virtual colonoscopy include its safety, high patient acceptance, and ability to provide a full structural evaluation of the entire colon.

Technique

Although a variety of scanning techniques have been described for virtual colonoscopy, the same basic imaging principles apply: cleansing the patient's colon using a standard barium enema or colonoscopy bowel preparation, colonic insufflation with room-air or carbon dioxide and thin-section helical CT of the abdomen and pelvis followed by off-line computer manipulation of the CT dataset to facilitate inspection of the colonic wall. All the methods described previously, including MPR, surface rendering and volume rendering, have been applied successfully to virtual colonoscopy and the various techniques have been found to be complementary. One clear consensus emerging from the various centres with prolonged experience in virtual colonoscopy is that the key feature of image review is the inspection of the 2D slices as the primary diagnostic method with 3D 'virtual views' reserved for problem solving.

Bowel preparation

Virtual colonoscopy requires a well-prepared, cleansed colon to achieve appropriate sensitivity and specificity. Retained stool can simulate polyps, decreasing specificity while retained fluid can obscure polyps, resulting in decreased sensitivity. The standard colonoscopy preparation (polyethylene glycol electrolyte solution, Go-Lytely; Braintree Laboratories, Braintree, MA) tends to result in more retained fluid than other preparations (magnesium citrate, bisacodyl tablets, cleansing enemas, or suppositories, Fleet 3 Prep kit, C.B. Fleet Co., Inc., Lynchburg, VA)[9]. At this time a full colon cleansing preparation is required to achieve acceptable results. Orally administered barium contrast products to mark or tag faecal residue are under investigation. The incentive behind the development of such products is to minimize bowel preparation requirements and increase patient compliance. The efficacy of these agents remains unproven, as shown by a study by Fletcher et al.[10], who found no benefit in using orally administered barium contrast prior to scanning.

Some investigators have suggested the use of a spasmolytic to prevent unwanted colonic collapse and spasm, a problem encountered most commonly in the sigmoid colon. However, the benefit of spasmolytic agents is controversial. No beneficial effect from routine glucagon administration with respect to colonic distension was seen in 60 patients who were scanned in the supine and prone positions[11]. Furthermore, as a result of its effect on the ileocaecal valve, glucagon can cause unwanted reflux of air into the small bowel and can secondarily reduce colonic distension.

CT scan acquisition

Typical single-detector CT imaging parameters[12] include a collimation of 5 mm or less, a table speed of 6.25 mm/s (pitch 1.25), 110 mA or lower, 110 kVp, and a 512×512 matrix. A single acquisition of the abdomen and pelvis is obtained with the patient breath-holding for the first 15–20 s of the scan (to cover the upper abdomen) while the remainder of the data is acquired during gentle respiration. Using multi-slice helical CT scanners the entire acquisition can be obtained in a single breath-hold using collimation of 2.5 mm, reconstruction index of 1–2 mm with similar mA and kVp used for single-slice scanners. Following the supine scan, the helical CT is routinely repeated with the patient prone. The use of both supine and prone helical CT datasets helps differentiate mobile stool from fixed pathology such as cancers and polyps, allows more even distension of the colon, and improves visualization of segments of colon obscured by intraluminal fluid[10,13]. Fletcher and colleagues found that the prone scan allows for better distension of the sigmoid colon in a significant number of cases[10]. A study including 50 cases[14] showed results inferior to other studies[10,12], presumably because patients were scanned in the supine position only and several lesions, notably in the rectum, were obscured by retained fluid.

Unlike fibre-optic colonoscopy, sedation is not required and patients are immediately discharged from the CT suite without the need for observation or recovery. The patients' ability to return to work or other activities of daily living is important when considering societal costs of colorectal cancer screening programmes. Considerable reduction in scanning time and motion artifact due to respiration has been achieved with new-generation multi-detector CT scanners. Preliminary results published by Rust et al.[15] show that utilizing virtual multi-slice CT colonoscopy, polyps and cancer of the colon can be reliably detected, if proper cleansing and distension is provided. On axial images alone smaller polyps may be assessed. The high z-axis resolution of MSCT offers superior conditions for CT-based virtual colonoscopy. Newer-generation CT scanners hold the promise of even greater speed and resolution than the current multislice CT scanners. Whether this new technology will result in greater accuracy is unknown.

Radiation dose

Hara et al.[16] reported that the radiation dose could be reduced by using the lower milli-amperage setting of 70 mA (5-mm collimation, 3-mm reconstruction interval, and a 1.3 pitch) compared with that of standard body CT settings (140 mA). They reported no change in the diagnostic efficacy between CT settings of 140 mA and 70 mA, while the effective dose equivalent for the acquisition of a single supine dataset was 1.87 mGy for men and 2.85 mGy for women. This dose would double by performing both prone and supine scanning. However, the doubling of dose still remains approximately 20% lower than the typical dose for double-contrast barium enema (4.53 mGy for men and 7.45 mGy for women)[16]. Mendelson and Forbes[17] reported a similar radiation dose, less than 5 mSv for the acquisition of supine and prone scans, compared with 8 mSv for conventional double-contrast barium enema.

Image display

Following image acquisition the CT data can be viewed using a variety of techniques[18–23]. These include simple evaluation of the axial CT images at lung window settings, multi-planar reformatted images and 3D endoluminal (simulating conventional endoscopy images) and extraluminal images (simulating barium enema images). Newer methods have used mathematically straightened views of the colon and mathematically 'unravelled' views of the colon (virtual gross pathology). The first method unfolds the colon as a straight tube, eliminating all physiological curves. The second method opens the colon along its longitudinal axis and is inspected in a flat rather than tubular form to simulate gross pathology. Which of these methods will prove to be the best in terms of speed and accuracy is, as yet, unclear. However, most investigators now agree that review of 2D images at lung window settings is sufficient for detection of potential abnormalities, and 3D post-processed views are necessary only for characterization of these potential lesions. The main role of the post-processed 3D views is to differentiate polyps from complex normal colonic folds which can have a similar appearance when viewed in profile using the axial images alone.

Macari et al.[24] compared the results of complete 2D and 3D CT colonography and conventional colonoscopy in detecting colorectal polyps in 42 patients. The authors concluded that axial 2D CT colonography (review of the axial slices) could be performed quickly and accurately. Furthermore, the authors concluded that results are not improved with the 3D virtual images. As computer processing techniques advance, complex image analysis software and computer-aided diagnosis may replace the current 'accepted' viewing techniques. In addition, expected improvements in CT data acquisition (8- and 16-channel multi-detector systems) are likely to improve test performance in the future as a result of shorter acquisition time, fewer image artifacts, and superior z-axis image resolution.

Role of MRI

Virtual endoscopy based on 3D MRI is also feasible and may also be an alternative to CT[25,26]. MRI methods are being pursued primarily as a way to eliminate the need for ionizing radiation. As in CT colonography, the images should be acquired in the prone and supine position. Image analysis is based on similar techniques used in CT-based methods, previously discussed. In a study[26] of 132 patients, MRI image quality was sufficient for diagnosis in 127 (96%) patients. Most small (5-mm diameter) masses were overlooked at magnetic resonance colonography (MRC), but 19 of 31 lesions of 6–10 mm, and 26 of 27 large (>10-mm) lesions were correctly identified. For these large masses, MRC had a sensitivity of 93%, specificity of 99%, positive predictive value of 92%, and negative predictive value of 98% for detection of masses. Pappalardo et al.[27] published a study on 70 consecutive patients and achieved a diagnostic accuracy similar to conventional colonoscopy (sensitivity 96%, specificity 93%, positive predictive value 98%, and negative predictive value 87.5%).

Faecal tagging to avoid colonic cleansing can be performed successfully in MRC[28]. The patients ingest 10 ml of a standard MRI contrast product (gadoterate meglumine) prior to three low-fibre meals. The lack of ionizing radiation is an advantage of MRC, although the use of a contrast fluid enema is a less appealing feature. Air may prove to be a more tolerable alternative in the future of MRC if technical challenges can be overcome.

Results of CT colonography

Preliminary results indicated that the accuracy of CT virtual colonoscopy for polyp detection exceeded barium enema and approached conventional colonoscopy. Hara et al.[29] of the Mayo Clinic evaluated 30 endoscopically proven polyps in 10 patients and detected 100% of all polyps greater than 1 cm in diameter, 71% of polyps between 0.5 and 0.9 cm and up to 28% of polyps smaller than 0.5 cm. In a subsequent study[30] the same group evaluated 70 consecutive patients and reported a sensitivity and specificity for patients with adenomatous polyps >10 mm of 75% and 90%, for patients with adenomatous polyps >5 mm the result was 66% and 63%, and for patients with adenomatous polyps <5 mm it was 45% and 80%, respectively. Dachman et al.[31], of the University of Chicago, using combined axial 2D CT images with limited 3D endoluminal reconstructions for problem-solving in 44 patients with 22 proven polyps, reported a sensitivity for virtual colonoscopy of 83% and a specificity of 100% for polyps 8 mm or larger.

Recent published studies from the Boston Medical Center and the Mayo Clinic reported results on larger patient populations. Fenlon et al.[12] prospectively studied 100 patients at high risk for colorectal neoplasia (60 men and 40 women; mean age 62 years). Virtual colonoscopy was performed immediately before conventional colonoscopy. The entire colon was visualized by virtual colonoscopy in 87 patients and by conventional colonoscopy in 89. Fifty-one patients had normal findings on conventional colonoscopy. In the remaining 49 patients a total of 115 polyps and three carcinomas were identified. Virtual colonoscopy identified all three cancers, 20 of 22 polyps that were 10 mm or more in diameter (91%), 33 of 40 that were 6–9 mm (82%), and 29 of 53 that were 5 mm or smaller (55%). There were 19 false-positive findings of polyps and no false-positive findings of cancer. Of the 69 adenomatous polyps, 46 of the 51 that were 6 mm or more in diameter (90%) and 12 of the 18 that were 5 mm or smaller (67%) were correctly identified by virtual colonoscopy. The authors concluded that, in patients at high risk for colorectal neoplasia, virtual and conventional colonoscopy have similar efficacy for the detection of polyps that are 6 mm or more in diameter. Fletcher et al.[10] published the largest series to date, including 180 patients with 420 colonoscopically proved polyps. These patients were known to have, or were suspected to have, colorectal neoplasm, except for 20 patients recruited from a surveillance population with a low prevalence of large polyps. By using supine and prone patient positioning the sensitivity and specificity for the identification of patients with polyps 1 cm or greater were 85% (82 of 96 patients) and 93% (78 of 84 patients), respectively. The sensitivity and specificity for the detection of polyps 5 mm or greater were 88% (114 of 130 patients) and 72% (36 of 50 patients), respectively. Other studies on smaller series have also been recently published, reporting similar results[32,33].

Proper technique is essential to achieving good results, as demonstrated by Fletcher et al.[10] and Fenlon et al.[12]. Results significantly improve if patients are scanned in prone and supine position and adequate colon distension is achieved. Retained fluid in the colon can be minimized with improvement in bowel preparation[9,10,12]. The study published by Pescatore et al.[14] suggests that scanning patients only in the supine position results in a decreased number of lesions detected, mainly because of retained fluid and a collapsed colon. As technical problems are solved the majority of false-negative studies will be attributable to perceptual errors. Perceptive errors can be reduced with observer experience and improvement in image display[22]. Pescatore et al.[14] found that there was a significant improvement in reader performance during the second half of their study of 50 patients. As reader experience improved the false-positive findings decreased after analysis of the first 24 patients. Specificity was very modest for patients 1–24 but considerably improved for patients 25–50. As is true for conventional colonoscopy, virtual colonoscopy has a substantial learning-curve process. Several major centres offer training fellowships as well as Internet-based tutorials in virtual colonoscopy (www.virtualcolonoscopy.net).

Indications for virtual colonoscopy

Occlusive carcinoma

Fenlon et al.[34] reported another application of virtual colonoscopy, the preoperative assessment of the colon proximal to an occlusive cancer (defined as a tumour that cannot be traversed endoscopically). In 29 patients with occlusive carcinomas, virtual colonoscopy identified all 29 occlusive cancers and demonstrated two cancers and 24 polyps in the proximal colon. Both of the synchronous cancers were confirmed intraoperatively and resected. Virtual colonoscopy successfully demonstrated the proximal colon in 26 of 29 patients studied, compared with preoperative barium enema that failed to adequately demonstrate the proximal colon in any patient studied. In three patients the retained stools proximal to an occlusive tumour prevented a complete virtual colonoscopic evaluation. Morrin et al.[35] had similar results, and found that CT colonography is superior to barium enema to assess the colon proximal to an occlusive tumour. A total of 97% (87/90) of all colonic segments were adequately visualized at CT colonography in patients with obstructing colorectal lesions (15 patients were referred after incomplete colonoscopy) compared with 60% (26/42) of segments at barium enema.

Incomplete colonoscopy

Colonoscopy fails to visualize the caecum in a significant number of patients; the completion rate may be 80–90% or less. Thiis-Evensen et al.[36] published their findings in a total of 241 men and women randomly selected from the population register who were offered a colonoscopic screening examination to detect and remove polyps. The caecum was intubated in only 193 (80%) of patients. More than half of the adenomas detected were localized proximal to the sigmoid colon and, in nearly half of the adenoma-bearing subjects examined, the adenoma was proximal to the descending colon. Nicholson and colleagues[37] reported a similar distribution of adenomas in 1131 asymptomatic individuals who underwent full colonoscopy. In 25% of people found to have adenomas, the adenomas were found only in the proximal colon. This emphasizes the importance of a screening method being able to view the entirety of the colon.

Virtual colonoscopy excels in the evaluation of the ascending colon, particularly the caecum, due to the degree of distension achievable and the typical lack of spasm or muscular hypertrophy that is seen in the sigmoid colon. It is therefore a useful complement to an incomplete colonoscopy[38,39]. Morrin et al.[38] prospectively studied 40 patients in whom the caecum could not be reached endoscopically despite adequate bowel preparation. CT colonography was performed within 2 h of incomplete colonoscopy in these 40 patients. In addition, 26 patients (65%) underwent barium enema immediately after CT colonography. CT colonography was better tolerated than barium enema. CT colonography adequately revealed 96% of all colonic segments; in comparison, barium enema adequately revealed 91% of all segments ($p < 0.05$).

Colon cancer screening

Decision processes regarding suitability of a test for screening are complex and involve estimates of performance characteristics, long-term outcomes, cost, patient acceptability, compliance and availability. The true diagnostic performance of virtual colonoscopy in a purely screening population has not yet been established and further studies such as the ongoing ACRIN, MUSC and European trials are awaited.

Virtual colonoscopy has been shown to be a safe test; none of the studies published so far has reported complications. It is also acceptable and well tolerated by patients. Patients can return to work immediately after the procedure, since no sedation is required.

Several papers[12,40–42] have addressed the place of virtual colonoscopy in the screening model of colon cancer. Adenomatous polyps are common, being present in 30–50% of persons over 50 years of age. Most measure less than 1 cm and, within this subset, the probability of malignancy is extremely low and the likelihood of any lesion progressing to malignancy is extremely small. Many non-neoplastic polyps also measure less than 1 cm. Because many small polyps have no malignant potential, it may be possible to target only polyps above a certain size threshold (6 mm or even 1 cm) for colon cancer screening and colonoscopic removal, and by doing so achieve benefits comparable to universal polypectomy, with considerable savings in cost and risk. There is a consensus among researchers that virtual colonoscopy has the ability to separate patients with colons containing only subcentimetre insignificant polyps or no polyps from patients with clinically significant polyps. Only the latter group would require therapeutic colonoscopy for polypectomy. As only 3–10% of average-risk persons age 50 years or over have a polyp 1 cm or greater in size, a test that could reliably and accurately identify this group would result in a dramatic reduction in the number of purely diagnostic colonoscopies performed, freeing up endoscopy services for those patients requiring therapeutic intervention.

Cost analysis assessments of virtual colonoscopy will have a major impact on its potential use for CRC screening. Such assessments are complex and must include analysis of basic costs for equipment, running costs, personnel training, staffing, technical and professional fees, as well as estimates of performance characteristics (in particular, the test's specificity), patient compliance rates, selected intervals for screening, cost of cancer treatment, and long-term outcomes. To be competitive, virtual colonoscopy will have to be provided at a cost only slightly greater than DCBE, and well below that of conventional colonoscopy.

Extracolonic findings

Since the entire abdomen and pelvis is scanned, the extracolonic organs can also be assessed. In 264 consecutive patients, Hara et al.[43] found 30 (11%) patients to have had highly important extracolonic findings, which resulted in further examinations in 18 (7%) patients, including ultrasonography in 10, CT in 13, and intravenous pyelography in one. Six patients underwent surgery because of incidentally discovered findings (two incidental abdominal aortic aneurysms greater than 4 cm, two asymptomatic renal adenocarcinomas, and one inguinal hernia-containing bowel). Almost half of all patients had abnormal extracolonic findings detected at CT colonography. No other colorectal screening examination has this advantage of detecting potentially life-threatening conditions, in an age group where those conditions have a higher prevalence.

CONCLUSIONS

The use of 3D imaging has previously been limited to major academic imaging departments and usually performed for research rather than clinical purposes. New applications in imaging have shown clear roles for 3D imaging for the detection and demonstration of pathology. By understanding the principles, indications, advantages and disadvantages of the various 3D techniques, radiologists and other physicians involved in imaging can capitalize on these emerging technologies. New workstations are now less expensive, less complicated, and are more available than ever before. One specific application of 3D imaging has been the emergence of virtual colonoscopy. Although the application of 3D imaging to create the virtual images simulating colonoscopy is likely to have been the reason for its initial appeal, most authorities now believe that the role of 3D processing in the detection of polyps is for problem-solving rather than detection.

References

1. Fleischmann D, Rubin G, Paik D et al. Stair-step artifacts with single versus multiple detector-row helical CT. Radiology. 2000;216:185–96.
2. Wong K, Paulson E, Nelson R. Breath-hold three-dimensional CT of the liver with multi-detector row helical CT. Radiology. 2001;219:75–9.
3. Baek S, Sheafor D, Keogan M, DeLong D, Nelson R. Two-dimensional multiplanar and three-dimensional volume-rendered vascular CT in pancreatic carcinoma: interobserver agreement and comparison with standard helical techniques. Am J Roentgenol. 2001;176:1467–73.
4. Hopper K, Iyriboz T, Wise S, Neuman J, Mauger D, Kasales C. Mucosal detail at CT virtual reality: surface versus volume rendering. Radiology. 2000;214:517–22.
5. Calhoun P, Kuszyk B, Heath D, Carley J, Fishman E. Three-dimensional volume rendering of spiral CT data: theory and method. Radiographics. 1999;19:745–64.
6. Katyal S, Oliver J, Buck D, Federle M. Detection of vascular complications after liver transplantation: early experience in multislice CT angiography with volume rendering. Am J Roentgenol. 2000;175:1735–9.
7. Hong K, Freeny P. Pancreaticoduodenal arcades and dorsal pancreatic artery: comparison of CT angiography with three-dimensional volume rendering, maximum intensity projection, and shaded-surface display. Am J Roentgenol. 1999;172:925–31.
8. Kondo H, Kanematsu M, Shiratori Y et al. MR cholangiography with volume rendering: receiver operating characteristic curve analysis in patients with choledocholithiasis. Am J Roentgenol. 2001;176:1183–9.
9. Fletcher JG, Johnson CD, MacCarty RL et al. CT colonography: overcoming problems of collapse and colonic fluid. Radiology. 1998;209(P):296 (abstract).
10. Joel G, Fletcher C, Johnson D et al. Optimization of CT colonography technique: prospective trial in 180 patients. Radiology. 2000;216:704–11.
11. Yee J, Hung RK, Akerkar GA, Wall SD. The usefulness of glucagon hydrochloride for colonic distention in CT colonography. Am J Roentgenol. 1999;173:169–72.
12. Fenlon HM, Nunes DP, Schroy PC 3rd, Barish MA, Clarke PD, Ferrucci JT. A comparison of virtual and conventional colonoscopy for the detection of colorectal polyps. N Engl J Med. 1999;341:1496–503.
13. Chen SC, Lu DS, Hecht JR, Kadell BM. CT colonography: value of scanning in both the supine and prone positions. Am J Roentgenol. 1999;172:595–9.
14. Pescatore P, Glucker T, Delarive J et al. Diagnostic accuracy and interobserver agreement of CT colonography: Gut. 2000;47:126–30.
15. Rust GF, Eisele O, Hoffmann JN, Kopp R, Furst H, Reiser M. [Virtual colonoscopy with multi-slice computerized tomography. Preliminary results]. Radiology. 2000;40:274–82.
16. Hara AK, Johnson CD, Reed JE et al. Reducing data size and radiation dose for CT colonography. Am J Roentgenol. 1997;168:1181–4.

17. Mendelson RM, Forbes GM. Virtually viewing the large bowel: the future of colorectal cancer screening? Med J Aust. 2000;172:416–17.
18. Summers RM, Beaulieu CF, Pusanik LM et al. Automated polyp detector for CT colonography: feasibility study. Radiology. 2000;216:284–90.
19. Paik DS, Beaulieu CF, Jeffrey RB Jr, Karadi CA, Napel S. Visualization modes for CT colonography using cylindrical and planar map projections. J Comput Assist Tomogr. 2000;24:179–88.
20. Wyatt CL, Ge Y, Vining DJ. Automatic segmentation of the colon for virtual colonoscopy. Comput Med Imaging Graph. 2000;24:1–9.
21. Sheppard DG, Iyer RB, Herron D, Charnsangavej C. Subtraction CT colonography: feasibility in an animal model. Clin Radiol. 1999;54:126–32.
22. Hopper KD, Iyriboz AT, Wise SW, Neuman JD, Mauger DT, Kasales CJ. Mucosal detail at CT virtual reality: surface versus volume rendering. Radiology. 2000;214:517–22.
23. Samara Y, Fiebich M, Dachman AH, Kuniyoshi JK, Doi K, Hoffmann KR. Automated calculation of the centerline of the human colon on CT images. Acad Radiol. 1999;6:352–9.
24. Macari M, Milano A, Lavelle M, Berman P, Megibow AJ. Comparison of time-efficient CT colonography with two- and three-dimensional colonic evaluation for detecting colorectal polyps. Am J Roentgenol. 2000;174:1543.
25. Luboldt W, Frohlich JM, Schneider N, Weishaupt D, Landolt F, Debatin JF. MR colonography: optimized enema composition. Radiology. 1999;212:265–9.
26. Luboldt W, Bauerfeind P, Wildermuth S, Marincek B, Fried M, Debatin JF. Colonic masses: detection with MR colonography. Radiology. 2000;216:383–8.
27. Pappalardo G, Polettini E, Frattaroli FM et al. Magnetic resonance colonography versus conventional colonoscopy for the detection of colonic endoluminal lesions. Gastroenterology. 2000;119:300–4.
28. Weishaupt D, Patak MA, Froehlich J, Ruehm SG, Debatin JF. Faecal tagging to avoid colonic cleansing before MRI colonography. Lancet. 1999;354:835–6.
29. Hara AK, Johnson CD, Reed JE et al. Detection of colorectal polyps by computed tomographic colography: feasibility of a novel technique. Gastroenterology. 1996;110:284–90.
30. Hara AK, Johnson CD, Reed JE, Ehman RL, Ilstrup DM. Colorectal polyp detection with CT colography: two- versus three-dimensional techniques (work in progress). Radiology. 1996;200:49–54.
31. Dachman AH, Kuniyoshi JK, Boyle CM et al. CT colonography with three-dimensional problem solving for detection of colonic polyps. Am J Roentgenol. 1998;171:989–95.
32. Kay CL, Kulling D, Hawes RH, Young JW, Cotton PB. Virtual endoscopy – comparison with colonoscopy in the detection of space-occupying lesions of the colon. Endoscopy. 2000;32:226–32.
33. Morra A, Meduri S, Ammar L, Ukmar M, Pozzi Mucelli R. [Colonoscopy with computed tomography with volume reconstruction. The results and a comparison with endoscopy and surgery]. Radiol Med (Torino). 1999;98:162–7.
34. Fenlon HM, McAneny DB, Nunes DP, Clarke PD, Ferrucci JT. Occlusive colon carcinoma: virtual colonoscopy in the preoperative evaluation of the proximal colon. Radiology. 1999;210:423–8.
35. Morrin MM, Farrell RJ, Raptopoulos V, McGee JB, Bleday R, Kruskal JB. Role of virtual computed tomographic colonography in patients with colorectal cancers and obstructing colorectal lesions. Dis Colon Rectum. 2000;43:303–11.
36. Thiis-Evensen E, Hoff GS, Sauar J, Majak BM, Vatn MH. Flexible sigmoidoscopy or colonoscopy as a screening modality for colorectal adenomas in older age groups? Findings in a cohort of the normal population aged 63–72 years. Gut. 1999;45:834–9.
37. Nicholson FB, Korman MG, Stern AI, Hansky J. Distribution of colorectal adenomas: implications for bowel cancer screening. Med J Aust. 2000;172:428–30.
38. Morrin MM, Kruskal JB, Farrell RJ, Goldberg SN, McGee JB, Raptopoulos V. Endoluminal CT colonography after an incomplete endoscopic colonoscopy. Am J Roentgenol. 1999;172:913–18.
39. Macari M, Berman P, Dicker M, Milano A, Megibow AJ. Usefulness of CT colonography in patients with incomplete colonoscopy. Am J Roentgenol. 1999;173:561–4.
40. Sonnenberg A, Delco F, Bauerfeind P. Is virtual colonoscopy a cost-effective option to screen for colorectal cancer? Am J Gastroenterol. 1999;94:2268–74.
    At this time, no data are available for reimbursement of virtual colonoscopy.

41. Chaoui AS, Blake MA, Barish MA, Fenlon HM. Virtual colonoscopy and colorectal cancer screening. Abdom Imaging. 2000;25:361–7.
42. Fenlon HM. Colorectal neoplasm detection using virtual colonoscopy: a feasibility study. Gastrointest Endosc. 2000;51:369–71.
43. Hara AK, Johnson CD, MacCarty RL, Welch TJ. Incidental extracolonic findings at CT colonography. Radiology. 2000;215:353–7.

Section V
Network systems

12
Training models – why and how?
S. BAR-MEIR

The concept of a simulator as a training tool is well established, notably in aviation[1,2]. Training pilots on simulators is being practised in order to avoid mistakes which may be critical and cost life. It is therefore only natural that simulators should also be used for training in the medical field. Performing an endoscopy requires skill and training. For each procedure there is a minimal number necessary to achieve competence. This ranges between 100 and 300 for procedures such as oesophagogastroduodenoscopy, colonoscopy and endoscopic retrograde cholangiopancreatography (ERCP)[3-6]. Many supervising physicians find that they have insufficient time to spend proctoring procedures. An endoscopic simulator, which saves time, would therefore be of value.

Historically the first endoscopic simulators were mechanical. Particular interest has focused on flexible sigmoidoscopy and colonoscopy[7,8]. The most advanced mechanical model available at the present time was developed by the university hospital of Tuebingen. This simulator consists of a reality-like phantom as regards dimension, colour, structure and tissue texture. It has a realistic and correct anatomy. This allows the simulation of all diagnostic and most of the therapeutic endoscopic interventions. It has an artificial tissue that enables the simulation of pathological findings such as strictures, polyps and tumours. It is also possible to perform therapeutic procedures such as polypectomy, ERCP with sphincterotomy, ablation of a tumour with laser or argon plasma coagulator and stent implantation. Unfortunately, this simulator has no interaction with the trainee, and the presence of a supervisor is required.

Animal models are more realistic, but they require continuous search for animals, and ethical objections are likely to limit their availability. It is for these reasons that the exteriorized dog colon used for colonoscopy[9] and the porcine models used for ERCP and sphincterotomy[10,11] have not gained popularity. Exceptions are the Erlangen models known as EASIE and the Enlarger Endo-Trainer in which the gastrointestinal tract and the pancreatico-biliary system are obtained from slaughtered pigs[12,13]. The ethical issue is eliminated because the pig gastrointestinal tract arrives from the slaughterhouse, where the animal is killed anyway for the supply of meat. Once available, the upper or lower gastrointestinal (GI) tract is installed on a plastic structure shaped like a human.

An ingenious perfusion system generates bleeding episodes. Erlangen models allow the performance of most GI procedures in a realistic fashion, very similar to humans. The only disadvantage of these models is the presence of two separate papillae for the biliary and pancreatic systems. The location of the biliary papilla is in the duodenal bulb 1 cm from the pylorus, thus allowing easy cannulation with a forward-view gastroscope. The papilla of the pancreatic duct is located 7–12 cm more distal in the duodenum and is considered difficult to cannulate.

In recent years computer-based simulators are becoming available[14,15]. The advantage of the computer-based simulator over an animal model is that it is always available with no need for earlier preparation. You just have to plug it into electricity and start training. At present there are two computer-based simulators of the GI tract, the GI-Mentor which was developed by Simbionix (Tel-Hashomer, Israel) and another one which was developed by Immersion Medical (Gaithersburg, Maryland). The Immersion simulator is suitable for diagnostic colonoscopy only. Steering and torque of the endoscope is possible and the sensation provided is very close to a real colonoscopy. The GI-Mentor of Simbionix allows diagnostic and therapeutic procedures including ERCP. The performance is on a mannequin with an authentic Pentax endoscope. Steering and torque of the endoscope is therefore possible, and suction and inflation buttons are also present. This device provides trainees with realistic sensations that mimic actual endoscopic examination. The simulator has a training programme that includes upper and lower GI cases and ERCP. Each case begins with a case history and allows trainees to practise examinations and operations appropriate for the case. Once a trainee has completed an assigned tutorial session the instructors can view the recorded events. Comments can be entered in the trainee file and special notes can be sent to the trainee using a message facility.

In two workshops held in 2000 in Nice (Francophone meeting) and in Hamburg (Endo club Nord), 71 gastroenterologists with experience in performing endoscopy for more than 1 year filled in an evaluation questionnaire following their work on the GI-Mentor[15]. Ninety-six per cent felt that the simulator met their expectations and 83% would consider it advantageous to be trained in an institution where such a simulator exists. Eighty-one per cent will use the simulator in their next training programme if it is available, and 90% felt that prior training on the GI-Mentor would reduce the potential risk to patients. The simulator was considered friendly by 97%, and 88% would recommend it to others.

At the present time there are only two small controlled trials where the value of the simulator in teaching endoscopy was assessed.

In the first study[16], five residents were assigned to a control group and five others to an experimental group. The last group trained on a sigmoidoscopy simulator before their first sigmoidoscopies on live patient volunteers. After 6–10 h training on the simulator the experimental group achieved a significantly faster insertion time (211 s versus 518 s) and a shorter mean length of examination (323 s versus 654 s). There was also a significant increase in the percentage of colon visualized (79% versus 45%) when compared with the control group.

In another study[17], fellows were divided into two groups of 11 each. The first group served as a control and the second group had 10 h training on the GI-Mentor. All fellows were asked to perform 20 upper GI endoscopies under tutoring. The simulator-pre-trained group required 18% less time to perform the procedure, 30% less assistance by tutor, and missed 8% less lesions.

Based on simulators already available the increased public awareness of medicolegal aspects, and the limited time of the supervising physicians, endoscopic training will be changed. Trainees will start their training on a computer-based simulator. More advanced training in therapeutic procedures will be obtained with the computer-based simulator first, and the Erlangen and Tuebingen models later. Such training will, most probably be, integrated into large training centres.

References

1. Helmreich RL, Foushee HC. Why crew resource management? In: Weiner EL, Kanki BG, Helmreich RL, eds. Cockpit Resource Management. San-Diego, CA: Academic Press, 1993;3–46.
2. Dusterberry JC. Introduction to simulation systems. Society of Photo-Optical Engineers 1975;59:141–2.
3. Farthing MJG, Walt RP, Allan RN et al. A national training program for gastroenterology and hepatology. Gut. 1966;38:459–70.
4. Anonymous. Methods of granting hospital privileges to perform gastrointestinal endoscopy. American Society for Gastrointestinal Endoscopy. Standards of training and practice committee. Gastrointest Endosc. 1992;38:765–7.
5. Tassios PS, Ladas SD, Grammenos I et al. Acquisition of competence in colonoscopy: the learning curve of trainees. Endoscopy. 1999;9:702–6.
6. Cass OH. Training to competence in gastrointestinal endoscopy: a plea for continuous measuring of objective end points. Endoscopy. 1999;9:751–4.
7. Rodining CB, Webb WR, Zingarelli WJ et al. Postgraduate surgical flexible endoscopic education. Ann Surg. 1986;203:272–4.
8. Bowman MA, Wherry DC. Training flexible sigmoidoscopy. Gastrointest Endosc. 1985;31:309–12.
9. Klua W, Knoch HG. Experimental phantoms for studying the colon. Z Gesamte Inn Med. 1984;39:197–9.
10. Naor MD. An established porcine model for animates training in diagnostic and therapeutic ERCP. Endoscopy. 1995;27:77–80.
11. Parasher VK, Toomey P, Clifton V et al. Simulated sphincterotomy in a pig model. Gastrointest Endosc. 1995;41:240–3.
12. Hochberger J, Neuman M, Maiss J et al. EASIE–Erlangen active simulator for interventional endoscopy – a new bio-simulation model – first experience gained in training workshops. Gastrointest Endosc. 1998;47:AB116.
13. Hochberger J, Maiss J, Magdeburg B, Hahn EG. Training simulators and education on gastrointestinal endoscopy: current status and perspectives in 2001. Endoscopy. 2001;33:1–8.
14. Bar-Meir S. Endoscopic simulator. Endoscopy. 2000;32:898–900.
15. Bar-Meir S. Endoscopic simulators: the state of art 2000. Gastrointest Endosc. 2000;52:701–3.
16. Tuggy ML. Virtual reality flexible sigmoidoscopy simulator training: impact on resident performance. J Am Board Fam Pract. 1998;11:426–33.
17. Fregonse D, Casetti T, Cestari R et al. Basic endoscopy training: usefulness of a computer-based simulator. Cooperative group for training in endoscopy. Gasrointest Endosc. 2001;S/AB 81.

13
The Minimal Standard Terminology for digestive endoscopy: introduction to structured reporting

M. DELVAUX

INTRODUCTION

Over the past decade the introduction of electronic endoscopes in the daily practice of digestive endoscopy has dramatically increased the possibilities of documenting endoscopic procedures with high-quality pictures. Combined with computers, the electronic endoscopes constitute actual 'endoscopic workstations'[1]. These workstations could then be linked to larger information systems (hospital information systems). However, this organization of the processing of data generated by endoscopic procedures supposes a standardization of the terms and image formats used. The advantages are that it is possible to search any database created, perform statistical analysis, and avoid the need for handwritten or typed reports. Around the world a considerable number of endoscopy record systems have been developed, but there has been no standardization of the terminology used. As a result a golden opportunity has been lost for sharing and comparing data collected from different centres.

The European Society for Gastrointestinal Endoscopy (ESGE) decided to resolve these issues. A Committee was established and included a number of experts from Belgium, France, Germany, Hungary, Italy, Spain and the United Kingdom. At an early stage it was felt important that the other world zones be represented, and representatives from the USA and Japan were co-opted into the Committee. Additionally, the three major endoscope manufacturers (Fujinon, Olympus and Pentax) and Normed-Verlag, the publisher of the OMED terminology, were invited to join the Committee as it was imperative that industry should be involved in this work as they were developing their own systems and compatibility between these was regarded as vital if the opportunities for sharing data were to be optimized. Between 1992 and 1993 a series of meetings of this Committee were held, concluding with a joint meeting of the ESGE group and the Computer Committee of the American Society for Gastrointestinal Endoscopy (ASGE). At this time the work was reviewed and modified, and the Committee was constituted as the Working Party for this report for the World Congresses of Gastroenterology and Digestive Endoscopy. A preliminary report was published during the Tenth World Congress of Gastroenterology and presented in Los Angeles[2].

AIMS

The major aim of the project was to devise a 'minimal' list of terms that could be included within any computer system used to record the results of a gastrointestinal endoscopic examination. At an early stage it was agreed not to attempt to develop a fully comprehensive terminology for computerization of endoscopic records. This attempt had been achieved in the past by the Terminology Committee of OMED (World Organization of Digestive Endoscopy) under the guidance of Z. Maratka[3]. This very detailed terminology was felt to be too complicated, and appeared to contain many double entries. However, the considerable contribution of this group was acknowledged and the structure of the new terminology was kept compatible with the existing one, offering the user the possibility of obtaining precise definitions of terms in the extended list.

To build this Minimal Standard Terminology (MST), it was decided that the terms selected must have wide acceptability and provide a means for recording the findings in the majority of examinations performed. Excessive detail was to be avoided and rare findings were to be recorded using 'free text' fields. Each term was selected on the basis that it would be expected to be used in at least 1 out of 100 consecutive examinations. The only terms included that did not fit this criterion were descriptive terms that could be found only in certain areas of the world (e.g. parasites), where they might be relatively common. In addition to the MST, the Committee addressed the issues of indications for endoscopic procedures and endoscopic diagnoses[4].

GENERAL PRINCIPLES

The MST is organized in three main sections (Figure 1), covering each type of endoscopic examination. When these procedures investigate several organs a separate list of terms has been provided for each. These lists are also subdivided into three main sections containing terms for description of:

1. *Reasons for performing an endoscopy.* Although a list of 'indications' is available in many countries, and is intended as a means of assessing the relevance and necessity for an endoscopic examination, this list had been devised on the basis of the appropriateness of an individual examination. While appreciating the reasons behind this decision the Committee felt that it was more important to record why a particular examination had been undertaken, rather than instruct users when an examination was acceptable. 'Reasons for' have, therefore, been divided into:
   (a) *Symptoms:* to allow a user to record the symptoms for which an endoscopic examination is required. This is particularly important when a disease is difficult to define.

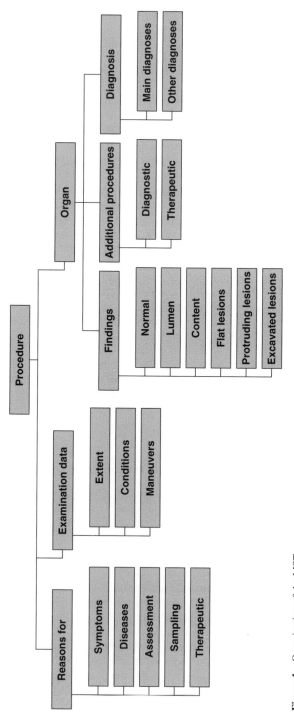

Figure 1 Organization of the MST

(b) *Diseases:* this lists the common diseases for which an endoscopic examination may be required. These can be qualified by 'Suspected...', 'For exclusion of ...', 'For follow-up of ...' or 'For therapy of...'.

(c) *Assessment of:* this category was introduced in the 'Reasons for' list in order to allow the recording of examinations performed to evaluate the status of a part of the gastrointestinal tract before or after a surgical procedure.

(d) *Diagnostic sampling:* this was included as a 'Reason for', as it was recognized that some examinations may be performed only to collect a sample.

3. *Endoscopic findings.* The terms selected are preceded, when applicable, by the OMED code number, as published in *Terminology, Definitions and Diagnostic Criteria in Digestive Endoscopy*, 4th edn[3]. A few 'terms' that were not originally included in the OMED classification were introduced because these words were in such common use that the Committee felt that they had to be included if the database created was to prove acceptable to an average user.

4. *Endoscopic diagnosis.* At the end of the list of terms for each examination there appears a list of diagnoses. This indicates a diagnosis that the endoscopist feels is most likely on the basis of macroscopic findings. This is not necessarily the final diagnosis, which takes into account the findings of any additional procedures performed, such as biopsy/cytology. The diagnostic list has been split into two parts: (i) main diagnoses, ordered by expected prevalence; (ii) other (rarer) diagnoses listed alphabetically. The decision as to on which list a particular diagnosis appears is based upon the expected frequency of this finding in a European context. This 'diagnosis' could be used to implement a 'conclusion' field within any report generated. Such a conclusion would be based on a synthesis of all of the findings recorded. This is particularly true when a number of different lesions are described, such as in inflammatory bowel diseases at colonoscopy. It is also recommended that it should be possible to record a 'negative conclusion' as well as a positive one. It is often as important to record that a feature is not present as it is to describe it; that is, for example, the failure to find any sign of bleeding when a patient presents with an apparent gastrointestinal bleed. It is suggested that it be possible to qualify a diagnosis by '*certain*', '*suspected*', '*probably not present*' and '*definitely excluded*'. At the end, a list of additional diagnostic (biopsies, cytology brushing, etc.) and therapeutic procedures is added.

ORGANIZATION OF THE LIST OF TERMS

The terms have been organized by examination type (Upper GI Endoscopy, Colonoscopy and ERCP), with an additional complementary list of Therapeutic Procedures that might be performed. Within each examination type the terms have been grouped under the various headings used within the OMED terminology for each organ examined (Table 1). There are a few exceptions to terms included under these headings. Most notable is the inclusion of post-surgical

Table 1 Major headings for grouping of terms in the structure of the MST

1.	Normal	Should be used if the organ has been entirely examined and everything is normal in it.
2.	Lumen*	Contains all terms regarding an abnormality in the size of the organ, any deformity, compression and evidence of previous surgery.
3.	Contents	Terms describing the presence of various materials within the organ.
4.	Mucosa	Terms describing patterns of the mucosa that are mainly diffuse and may involve all the mucosa of one limited area. These terms are not applicable to individual lesions.
5.	Flat lesions	Terms to be used for individual lesions which remain in the plane of the mucosa.
6.	Protruding lesions	Terms to be applied to lesions growing above the plane of the mucosa.
7.	Excavated lesions	Terms to be applied to lesions whose surface is beneath the plane of mucosa.

* This heading also includes some terms classified under 'Wall' in the OMED terminology.

findings under the 'Lumen' heading. Whilst this is not a 'lesion', it is apparent that the changes visible after a previous surgical procedure will be seen while examining the lumen of a particular organ (e.g. an ileocolonic anastomosis while examining the colon or a Billroth II anastomosis when within the stomach) and should be recorded at this time.

The list of terms displayed for any location varies with the organ being examined. For example, the term 'oesophagitis' appears only in the oesophageal section, while the term 'spot' is found in the stomach and colon but not in the oesophagus. Thus the list of terms is varied where a particular term is felt to be inappropriate for a particular location. Terms used to describe functional changes, such as contractility and elasticity of the wall, increased or decreased peristalsis, functional narrowing or extrinsic distortion, have been excluded from the minimal terminology as they were considered to be too subjective and imprecise to aid making a diagnosis. In addition, these terms were too open to misinterpretation for use in any multicentre studies.

When appropriate, each term has attached to it qualifying attributes which provide additional detail. The attributes are a list of descriptive terms such as size, number, extent, etc. for which there are a series of values appropriate to that term. For example, the attributes for a duodenal ulcer include: size (in millimetres); shape (superficial, cratered or linear); bleeding (yes, no or 'stigmata of recent bleeding', defined by Forrest's criteria). Every lesion described is placed in its location by the use of a list of sites relevant to the organ being examined.

TESTING AND MAINTENANCE OF THE MINIMAL STANDARD TERMINOLOGY

An initial retrospective testing has been performed at six centres, by matching MST terms with those currently in use in these centres. Some of the tests were performed with the original English version of the minimal terminology; however, most of the centres used a close translation of this terminology to their native language. These tests, including more than 10 000 cases, have indicated that the MST accurately described an average of 87% of 'reasons for', 94% of

TERMINOLOGY FOR DIGESTIVE ENDOSCOPY

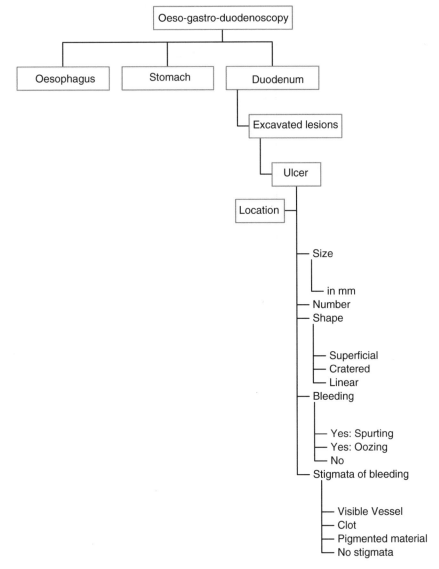

Figure 2 Structure of the links between terms and attributes

findings and 91% of 'endoscopic diagnosis'. The remaining findings required the use of free text (Table 2). However, the variation in the kinds of systems available for documentation in these centres did not allow for the recording of all the data needed to build a full endoscopic record. This also applies to the number of 'normal' findings, which in some of the studies were not recorded. The results are therefore related either to the sum of the pathological findings, or to the total of examinations.

Table 2 Number of examinations fully described using terms originally in the MST Results of the European Testing (Gaster Project)

	EGD			Colonoscopies			ERCP		
	No. of exams	Fully described	Percentage	No. of exams	Fully described	Percentage	No. of exams	Fully described	Percentage
Reasons for	2974	2680	90.1	1520	1376	90.5	739	707	95.6
Findings	3447	3436	99.7	1743	1729	99.2	1042	1031	99.0
Endoscopic diagnosis	2890	2813	97.3	1462	1375	94.0	714	669	93.7
Additional diagnostic procedures	1605	1603	99.8	458	458	100	74	59	79.7
Additional therapeutic procedures	163	153	93.8	226	220	97.3	403	378	93.8

In a second phase, prospective testing trials were undertaken, both in Europe and in the USA. In Europe the GASTER project, funded by the European Commission (DGXIII – Telematics) involved 11 university hospitals in various countries, that used a dedicated software, enabling recording of endoscopic cases with the MST and statistical analysis of free-text blocks[5]. Six thousand two hundred and thirty-two reports were analysed, comprising 3447 gastroscopies, 1743 colonoscopies and 1042 ERCPs. Overall, terms originally contained in the MST could describe fully 91.0% of all examinations where 'Reasons for' were described, 99.5% of examinations where 'findings' were described, 95.8% of all examinations containing descriptions of 'endoscopic diagnosis', 98.9% of examinations containing descriptions of 'additional diagnostic procedures' and 94.8% of examinations containing descriptions of 'additional therapeutic procedures'. Free text fields were only used in the other cases (less than 5% of cases on average). The detailed results of this testing are reported in Table 3. However, these excellent results must be analysed, taking into account the fact that many examination reports contained more than one description in each of the fields. So we performed a second statistical analysis that took into account the number of descriptions instead of the number of examinations. The results of this analysis are reported in Table 3.

The results of these tests have been used for updating and improving the MST. Hence, after the version 1.0 of the MST was published in 1996[4], the second version of the MST was published in 2000[6]. Moreover, it is accessible and can be downloaded from a number of web sites owned by the Gaster project (www.gaster.org), the ESGE (www.esge.com), the ASGE (www.asge.org) and the OMED (www.omed.org). On the last site, translation of the MST is provided in 10 languages.

ADVANTAGES OF THE USE OF THE MST FOR THE EDITION OF ENDOSCOPIC REPORTS

The use of a structured language for the edition of endoscopic reports request from users, i.e. endoscopists, an effort to become familiar with the structure of that language and modify their behaviour, in order to transfer the global concepts they build in natural language into a set of elemental data. This action of splitting of the data into elements requires the design of data models that will meet the actual situations where users are working.

The modelling of a structured language as a basis for standardization

An endoscopy report can be thought of as a file which contains a series of documents defined by the needs of practice and filled in with the data generated during a procedure. A standardization process of these data supposes that all the data elements that can be potentially introduced in an endoscopic report are taken into consideration and integrated in the model. On the other hand, a model integrating these data elements must be comprehensive for the user, as the data must be introduced in a logical way in the database and then retrieved to build

Table 3 Number of descriptions described using terms originally in the MST Results of the European Testing (Gaster Project)

	EGD			Colonoscopies			ERCP		
	No. of descriptions	Fully described	Percentage	No. of descriptions	Fully described	Percentage	No. of descriptions	Fully described	Percentage
Reasons for	4125	3499	84.8	2076	1745	84.1	1267	1125	88.8
Findings	11803	11448	97.0	2901	2790	96.2	4267	4023	94.3
Endoscopic diagnosis	7180	6803	94.7	1821	1611	88.5	2068	1615	78.1
Additional diagnostic procedures	1856	1850	99.7	505	497	98.4	110	89	80.9
Additional therapeutic procedures	178	166	93.3	260	252	96.9	691	638	92.3

up the report. Therefore, when all the data elements have been identified, one must create a coherent grouping of these elements. The MST lists provide these data elements. However, they need to be organized in logical way. As DICOM (Digital Imaging and Communication in Medicine) has integrated all data elements related to medical images in a standardized list of fields[7], we attempted to utilize a similar interdependent message/terminology architecture. This effort should result, in a near future, in the SNOMED-DICOM microglossary for digestive endoscopy that will enable the creation of templates for the content of the endoscopic report and thereby suggest value-sets for the coded entry of the various fields of the report[8]. This structuration of the data presupposes a detailed analysis of the data elements and their mutual relationship. Based on the results of this analysis, the model can be proposed as a logical integration of the data along the pathway that should be followed by the endoscopist building a report in natural language (Figure 3).

Using such a structured language offers the possibility of integration of all the data elements in an 'object', i.e. a set of data that is organized in a rigid structure

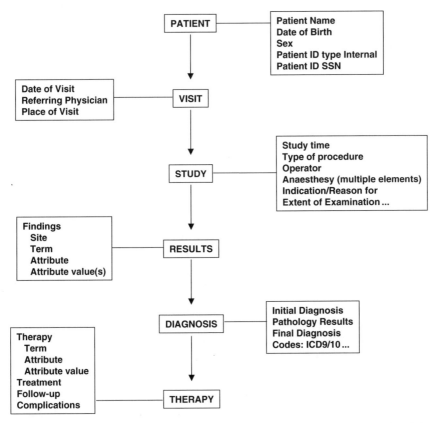

Figure 3 Example of an 'object' describing the visit of a patient in the endoscopy unit and the procedure that was performed

which can be shared and understood by different systems. These objects can then be easily transferred from one system to another one. Moreover, these objects can be easily retrieved from databases as relational databases currently used in medical informatics are more and more built as 'object-oriented' databases. Another advantage is a consequence of this architecture of the databases: data can be retrieved as structured subsets in a fast and secure process.

Clinical benefits for the use of a structured language

Although advances in endoscope technology have allowed the production of high-quality video images to be transmitted, captured and stored by modern, high-speed integrated circuits, image documentation and reporting has not progressed so fast. However, the constant increase in the use of computers for management of medical data has induced a strong need for the standardization of the data to be exchanged. Standardization means the coding of the data in a common format that can be read by multiple information systems, operated on different platforms. This goal is achieved by actions such as the DICOM or HL-7, as mentioned earlier, but also goes far beyond the medical needs: image formats such as JPEG, TGA and TIFF have been developed for purposes other than medicine. However, a medical image without the relevant associated data is of no value[9]. Thus the need for standardization of medical text data has become stronger over the past decade.

However, exchange of medical data supposes their mutual understanding between users at both ends of the chain along which exchange will occur: this statement encompasses the standardization of definitions of terms, the multilingual approach to terms and descriptions and the suitability of data to the clinical situation. This very important issue can be addressed in a proper way only by intensive testing of any standard system in actual clinical settings. Prospective trials must be undertaken for validation of the standards. In turn these standards, when used for clinical research, will enable cooperative studies, large outcome research protocols and quality assurance processes.

The use of structured reports in endoscopy, based on a structured language such as the MST, will allow statistical analysis of the databases based not only on the coded data using rigid coding systems, such as ICD, but the complete set of available data. Indeed, in a database structured with the MST, not only can the terms themselves be analysed but the attributes and attribute values can also be counted. Analysis of the data will thus be more detailed. The advantage for clinical research is obvious: standardization of the data in digestive endoscopy will support multicentre trials, will overcome the problems of multilingual data recording in cooperative studies and will promote outcome research. The latter point will become very important in the near future. Advances will be obtained only by analysis of large sets of data and will be based on evaluation of the following features: (a) suitability of data descriptions to observations, (b) measurement of appropriateness of diagnostic and therapeutic decisions made for the patient, (c) precise description of technical approaches to diseases, and (d) multidisciplinary understanding and management of the diseases. All these actions need an integration of medical data, at the level of each specialty in a first step but also an export of data from the specialized unit, i.e. the endoscopy unit, to the integrated care unit, through the hospital information system. Large standardized systems have failed in the past to cover medical data as a whole. This justifies the approach of the SNOMED to now promote the validation of microglossaries in specialty-related domains and to integrate these microglossaries at an upper level, making them interoperable by a common structure[10].

Future trends and maintenance of the MST

The future is represented by two main lines of action: one will be devoted to the maintenance of the MST with respect to evolution of knowledge and practice and to its preservation from inconsistent changes induced by a wider use. The second one will ensure the flexibility of the MST and its possible adaptation to specific situations.

Maintenance of the MST is a long-standing activity that must be integrated in the frame of a scientific society and, on the other hand, it must be an open process that will ensure fair responsiveness to new features. Recently the representatives of OMED, ESGE and ASGE have met and decided, with the cooperation of some Japanese colleagues, to set up an Editorial Board for the MST. This Board will have an international dimension and will care for the tasks related to MST, in close cooperation with the various scientific societies. The MST Editorial Board will be responsible for the maintenance of the versions of MST, the adaptation of it to new practice and the release of versions. The main task of the Board, besides its administrative tasks, will be to promote the use of the MST and to establish relationships with the National Societies for Gastrointestinal Endoscopy, supporting the production of accurate translations in the national languages and the organization of educational events to teach the community with the use of MST. Moreover, the Editorial Board will disseminate the MST among software developers and persuade them to implement it in their applications. In this way the Editorial Board will produce guidelines for writing a conformance statement that could be used by software developers to obtain a recognition that they properly implemented the MST. This would actually support its dissemination.

On the other hand, the MST must remain a living and evolving system. It must be able to adapt to local needs or to particular aspects of the practice. The prevalence of some digestive disorders varies from country to country. Techniques used in the limited area of one disease may appear useful in other conditions. The level of detail of the information contained in the report may be higher than the one fixed in the MST in some situations: cooperative studies on a specific topic may require additional information that was not required as the minimal set of data that should be described in any endoscopic report; local prevalence of a disease may justify some specific descriptions in some areas, etc. To solve these problems the MST should in the future be organized on the same basis as SNOMED is organizing microglossaries. This means that, besides the backbone of the MST, the current list of terms, one should be allowed to develop secondary lists of terms and/or attributes that would describe a given pathology in a more detailed way. To maintain the compatibility of these more detailed versions of the MST with the original one, each detailed list should refer to an existing term of the MST and it would be agreed that the exchange of data would take into account either the headline in the original MST or the complete set of descriptions for a particular type of findings, depending on the setting. In this case the structure of the MST would not be altered, and an extended list of terms would be transferred with reference to the original term, to which it would belong.

CONCLUSION

The Minimal Standard Terminology proposes a set of terms describing the various elements of the endoscopic report in a standardized way. These terms have been selected by a long process, and the lists have been tested in real clinical settings during all phases of development. This gives the community an outstanding opportunity to use a common language to describe endoscopic findings and to undertake multicentre trials. Using this common terminology will also support the connection of the endoscopic unit with the hospital information system, and the development of applications promoting the interoperability of information systems in digestive endoscopy. Taken together with the development of computerized imaging techniques, this will result in better documentation of endoscopic procedures and thereby in a considerable increase in the quality of the practice.

References

1. Delvaux M. Image management: the viewpoint of the clinician. Gastroenterologist. 1996;4:3–5.
2. Crespi M, Delvaux M, Schapiro M, Venables C, Zwiebel F. Minimal standards for a computerized endoscopic database. Am J Gastroenterol. 1994;89:S144–53.
3. Maratka Z. Terminology, Definitions and Diagnostic Criteria in Digestive Endoscopy, 4th edn. Bad Homburg, Germany: Normed Verlag, 1994.
4. Crespi M, Delvaux M, Schapiro M, Venables C, Zwiebel F. Working party report by the Committee for Minimal Standards of Terminology and Documentation in Digestive Endoscopy of the European Society of Gastrointestinal Endoscopy. Minimal Standard Terminology for a Computerized Endoscopic Database. Am J Gastroenterol. 1996;91:191–216.
5. Delvaux M, Crespi M, Armengol-Miro JR et al. Minimal Standard Terminology for Digestive Endoscopy: Prospective testing and validation in the GASTER project. Endoscopy. 2000;32:345–55.
6. Minimal Standard Terminology for Digestive Endoscopy, Version 2.0. International Editor: M. Delvaux, Endoscopy. 2000;32:159–88.
7. Digital imaging and communication in medicine (DICOM), NEMA PS3.1–PS3.12. The National Electrical Manufacturers' Association, Rosslyn, VA, 1992, 1993, 1995, 1997.
8. Digital imaging and communication in medicine (DICOM), NEMA PS3 Supplement 23: Structured reporting. The National Electrical Manufacturers' Association, Rosslyn, VA, 1997.
9. Brown NJG, Britton KE, Plummer DL. Standardisation in medical image management. Int J Med Inform. 1998;48:227–38.
10. Korman LY, Delvaux M, Bidgood D. Structured reporting in gastrointestinal endoscopy: integration with DICOM and Minimal Standard Terminology. J Med Inform. 1998;48:201–6.

Section VI
Ultrasound

14
Ultrasound in diffuse liver disease

L. BOLONDI, S. GAIANI, N. CELLI and F. PISCAGLIA

INTRODUCTION

The diagnosis of cirrhosis is currently based on percutaneous liver biopsy, although this procedure involves discomfort, costs of hospitalization, a 2–4% risk of complications[1,2] and may give rise to false negative results.

Non-invasive diagnostic tests for cirrhosis, alternative to liver biopsy, would therefore represent a major advance in these patients. Ultrasound (US) has been compared with liver biopsy for several years, with an overall accuracy of 70–75% and, relevant to advancements in US equipment, prospective studies pointing out detailed US features have been reported[3–5].

The ultrasonographic study of patients with diffuse liver disease includes the assessment of the following parameters: changes in liver morphology, surface nodularity, and altered echo-pattern.

LIVER MORPHOLOGY

Liver morphology may assist in the diagnosis of diffuse liver disease, particularly in cirrhosis, as the liver tends to shrink according to the progression of cirrhosis. In addition, due to the independent vascularization, the left and caudate lobes may become hypertrophic, occupying a relatively large proportion of the liver volume. The caudate-to-right lobe may therefore be useful to identify patients with cirrhosis with a specificity of 100% and a sensitivity of 84% using a cut-off of 0.65. The accuracy of this parameter may, however, change in cirrhosis of different aetiology, being lower for alcoholic diseases than in cases of virus-related and particularly HBV-related cirrhosis[6].

SURFACE NODULARITY

Surface nodularity is considered a specific sign of cirrhosis, and corresponds to the detection of regenerative nodules separated by fibrous scars at US. This sign

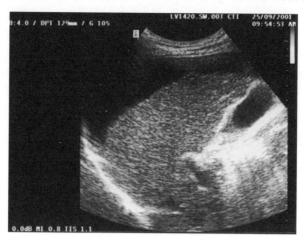

Figure 1 Nodular surface of the right lobe of the liver is better detected in the presence of ascites. Right intercostal scan

is easy to detect in the presence of ascites which better delineates the liver surface (Figure 1); otherwise it can be identified by careful examination of the inferior surface of the liver, especially in relation to the gallbladder and right kidney. The sensitivity of surface nodularity is relatively low (50% in the case of macronodular cirrhosis and 40% in the case of micronodular pattern), and it can be increased (up to 84%) by using a higher frequency 7.5 MHz probe. The specificity of this sign is very high (98%)[7].

ECHO PATTERN

The echo pattern of diffuse liver disease may include an increased reflectivity with a concomitant loss of definitions of portal vein walls, without a significant increase in attenuation, with fine and even echoes (bright liver) (Figure 2), while in the case of cirrhosis the echo texture is usually coarse and irregular. The lack of attenuation of the US beam may be useful in distinguishing fibrosis by fatty infiltration. However, this differentiation may be scarcely relevant from a practical point of view, as the two conditions may coexist, particularly in the case of alcoholic liver disease. In virus-related chronic liver disease, without evidence of fatty infiltration at pathological examination, the presence of bright liver is correlated with the severity of fibrosis. In conclusion, the coarse echo pattern, if associated with clinical and laboratory typical findings, is diagnostic for liver cirrhosis, with a sensibility relatively low (50%), but with a high specificity (90%)[8].

DIAGNOSIS

The diagnosis of liver cirrhosis may be supported by the detection of Doppler US findings related to portal hypertension, including the increase in calibre with

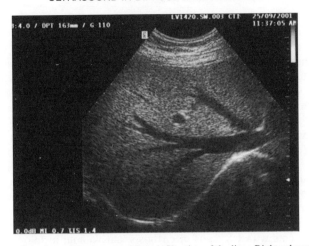

Figure 2 Increased echogenicity in case of fatty infiltration of the liver. Right subcostal scan

decrease of flow velocity of the portal vein, the presence of spontaneous portosystemic collaterals and ascites.

Several studies have reported wide variations in the normal limits of portal vein diameter (10–16 mm), that may be influenced by many factors, such as respiration, postural changes and postprandial state. In patients with advanced cirrhosis and portal hypertension a value of 15 mm offers a high specificity, but it is less sensitive. A value of 12 mm may be useful to differentiate chronic hepatitis from compensated cirrhosis[9]. The lack of variation in calibre during respiration in the splenic and superior mesenteric veins has been reported as a sensitive and highly specific sign of portal hypertension[10].

The main intrahepatic portal branches may be also dilated in portal hypertension, whereas the peripheral intrahepatic branches appear narrowed and tortuous, due to parenchymal fibrosis and nodular regeneration. Varying degrees of dilation of the splenic and superior mesenteric veins have been reported, and the upper limit ranges from 10 to 12 mm. Splenomegaly is usually associated with dilation of the splenic vein radicles, of the splenic vein and splenic artery. The upper normal limits for the spleen, evaluated with an intercostal scan crossing the hilum, are 12 mm for bipolar diameter and 45 cm^2 for the section area.

The detection of spontaneous portosystemic shunt is a specific sign of portal hypertension. The recanalized umbilical vein is easy to visualize as it runs within the ligamentus teres in the left lobe of the liver, particularly using colour Doppler that shows hepatofugal flow pathognomonic for portal hypertension. Other collaterals, such as the left gastric vein and retroperitoneal veins around the pancreas, may be more difficult to visualize because of intestinal gas. Large splenorenal shunts, connecting splenic varices with the left renal vein, may relieve portal hypertension. They appear as tortuous vessels near the lower pole of the spleen. Finally, the Doppler qualitative parameters (presence of portal thrombosis, identified for the presence of echoic material within the vessel or the signal absence at colour Doppler, and reversal portal flow), quantitative parameters (low value of portal flow velocity) and semiquantitative parameters (increased arterial impedance indexes in splenic and hepatic arteries) are useful for diagnosis.

Ultrasound has been compared with liver biopsy for several years, with an overall accuracy of 70–75% and, relative to advancements in US equipment, prospective studies pointing out detailed US features have been reported[3–5].

The accuracy of a US score model in predicting the final diagnosis in 212 patients with compensated chronic liver disease has been recently investigated[9]. Taking biopsy as criterion standard the US score, derived from liver, spleen and portal vein features, differed significantly between chronic hepatitis and cirrhosis (39 ± 33 vs. 100 ± 35; $p < 0.0001$). Discriminant analysis identified liver surface nodularity and portal flow velocity as independently associated with the diagnosis of cirrhosis ($p < 0.005$) and a score based on these two variables correctly identified cirrhosis in 82.2% of cases. In addition, this diagnostic model was able to identify cirrhosis even in the absence of typical histological patterns, as eight out of 32 patients with US signs of cirrhosis, but without histological cirrhosis, developed signs of decompensated cirrhosis during a 6-month follow-up.

Preliminary data on the use of US contrast agent to differentiate cirrhosis from non-cirrhotic liver disease based on transit-time analysis in the hepatic veins have been recently reported, and could provide new insight in the future[11].

CONCLUSION

US is accurate in diagnosing cirrhosis and may identify cirrhosis even in the absence of a typical histopathological pattern. However, neither percutaneous liver biopsy nor US can be assumed as the definite criterion standard for the diagnosis of compensated cirrhosis. Clinical, biochemical, and endoscopic parameters may be combined with US to further increase the reliability of a non-invasive diagnosis of cirrhosis.

References

1. Piccinino F, Sagnelli E, Pasquale G, Giusti G. Complications following percutaneous liver biopsy. A multicentre retrospective study on 68,276 biopsies. J Hepatol. 1986;2:165–73.
2. Lindor KD, Bru C, Jorgensen RA et al. The role of ultrasonography and automatic-needle biopsy in outpatient percutaneous liver biopsy. Hepatology. 1996;23:1079–83.
3. Sanford NL, Walsh P, Matis C, Baddeley H, Powell LW. Is ultrasonography useful in the assessment of diffuse parenchymal liver disease? Gastroenterology. 1985;89:186–91.
4. Saverymuttu SH, Joseph AE, Maxwell JD. Ultrasound scanning in the detection of hepatic fibrosis and steatosis. Br Med J. 1986;292:13–15.
5. Joseph AE, Saverymuttu SH, al-Sam S, Cook MG, Maxwell JD. Comparison of liver histology with ultrasonography in assessing diffuse parenchymal liver disease. Clin Radiol. 1991; 43:26–31.
6. Harbin WP, Rabert MJ, Ferrucci JT Jr. Diagnosis of cirrhosis based on regional changes in hepatic morphology. A radiological and pathological analysis. Radiology. 1980;136:717–23.
7. Di Lelio A, Cestari C, Lomazzi A, Beretta L. Cirrhosis: diagnosis with sonographic study of the liver surface. Radiology. 1989;172:389–92.
8. De Bongie JC, Pauls C, Fievez M, Wibin E. Prospective evaluation of the diagnostic accuracy of liver ultrasonography. Gut. 1981;22:130.

9. Gaiani S, Gramantieri L, Venturoli N *et al*. What is the criterion for differentiating chronic hepatitis from compensated cirrhosis? A prospective study comparing ultrasonography and percutaneous liver biopsy. J Hepatol. 1997;27:979–85.
10. Bolondi L, Gandolfi L, Arienti V *et al*. Ultrasonography in the diagnosis of portal hypertension: diminished response of portal vessels to respiration. Radiology. 1982;142:167–72.
11. Albrecht T, Blomley MJ, Cosgrove DO *et al*. Non-invasive diagnosis of hepatic cirrhosis by transit-time analysis of an ultrasound contrast agent. Lancet. 1999;353:1579–83.

15
Use of ultrasound contrast agents in hepatology

A. K. P. LIM, C. J. HARVEY, S. D. TAYLOR-ROBINSON,
M. J. K. BLOMLEY and D. O. COSGROVE

INTRODUCTION

Ultrasound, unlike all other imaging modalities, has until relatively recently, lacked effective contrast agents. This, however, was rectified with the introduction of microbubbles which have revolutionized the field[1,2]. The purpose of this article is to give an overview of the general principles of imaging with microbubbles and their applications within the liver.

MICROBUBBLES

Microbubbles range between 2 and 7 μm in diameter, traverse capillaries and are safe effective echo enhancers[3]. Levovist (SHU 508A; Schering AG, Germany), the most commonly used agent, is licensed in many countries and consists of galactose microcrystals whose surfaces provide nidation sites on which air bubbles form when they are suspended in water[4]. These bubbles are stabilized by a trace of palmitic acid which acts as a surfactant, thus allowing the pulmonary circulation to be crossed. However, these microbubbles are only stable and effective for up to 20 min. Thus, newer more-stable agents with heavier-molecular-weight gases and stronger coating membranes have been developed. This has resulted in prolonged enhancement times. Examples include Sonovue (Bracco, Milan, Italy) and Definity (Dupont Merck, Billerica, MA, USA) which utilise sulphur hexafluoride and perfluoropropane gases respectively[5]. Their membranes are more stable with the use of phospholipids. A cyanoacrylate coat has also been utilized to provide a firmer surrounding shell, e.g. Sonavist (SH U 563A, Schering AG, Germany)[6].

MICROBUBBLE IMAGING MODES

The interactions of microbubbles with an ultrasound beam are complex. Since a microbubble is more compressible than soft tissue, when it is exposed to an oscillating acoustic signal, alternate expansion and contraction occurs. At low acoustic power, these oscillations are equal and symmetrical (linear behaviour) and the frequency of the scattered signal is unaltered with the scattering intensity linearly related to that of the incident beam. As the acoustic power increases, more complex non-linear interactions occur as the expansion and contraction phases become unequal because the microbubbles resist compression more strongly than expansion. The microbubbles then behave like a musical instrument emitting harmonic signals at multiples of the insonating frequency. These emitted harmonic signals are microbubble specific and may be regarded as a signature of that agent. At still higher powers (although within accepted limits for diagnostic imaging), highly non-linear behaviour occurs with disruption or scintillation which may be imaged by a number of modes (see below). Vascularity (blood pool phase) of focal liver lesions can be imaged at low power to minimize bubble destruction, whilst uptake of the contrast agent within the lesion can be assessed by disruption of the bubbles using high power and imaged using the methods described below.

FOCAL LIVER LESIONS (VASCULAR PHASE)

Contrast-enhanced imaging of focal liver lesions can be performed during the vascular phase assessing the dynamic enhancement pattern and the vascular morphology of the lesion. This has proved particularly useful in diagnosis of haemangiomas because, despite their vascular nature, the blood flow within a haemangioma is too slow to be detected by conventional Doppler modes. After administration of ultrasound contrast agents, peripheral globular enhancement can be demonstrated, followed by the classic delayed centripetal in filling typical of haemangiomas. These characteristics are analogous to that seen on computed tomography (CT) and magnetic resonance imaging (MRI)[7,8]. The presence of hypervascularity in a lesion is non-specific and can be seen in focal nodular hyperplasic (FNH), hepatocellular carcinomas (HCC) or vascular metastases (e.g. neuroendocrine tumours). In these cases, combination with late/liver-specific phase scanning is more helpful (see below).

Another useful application of assessing lesions in the vascular phase is to look for evidence of viable tumour after ablative therapy. Choi and colleagues[9] studied 40 patients with HCCs which were treated with radio-frequency ablation and assessed their vascularity with microbubble-enhanced Doppler ultrasound. Six patients showed signal enhancement in the vascular phase in the treated regions suggesting residual or recurrent disease. The residual tumours were later confirmed on CT scan.

FOCAL LIVER LESIONS (LATE/LIVER-SPECIFIC PHASE)

Some contrast agents have a late liver-specific phase where the bubbles accumulate in normal liver parenchyma 2–5 min after injection when the vascular enhancement has faded. This is analogous to liver-specific contrast agents used in MRI[10] and is particularly useful for lesion detection and characterization. Microbubbles known to exhibit liver-specific behaviour are Levovist[11–13], Sonovist (both Schering AG, Germany)[11], Sonazoid (NC100100; Nycomed Amersham, Norway)[14] and BR14 (Bracco SPA, Italy)[15]. The mechanism of hepatic uptake is not completely understood. Mediation by the reticuloendothelial system, pooling or endothelial adherence in the liver sinusoids of the microbubbles have been postulated as mechanisms. For some agents (Sonavist), Kupffer cell up-take has been demonstrated[16].

Late-phase imaging requires microbubble-specific non-linear imaging techniques, such as colour stimulated acoustic enhancement (SAE), agent detection imaging (ADI) or phase inversion mode (PIM). In SAE, bubble inactivation produces transient echoes resulting in phase change between Doppler pulses and are interpreted as a Doppler shift. ADI also utilises this mechanism but with improved technical innovation resulting in improved spatial resolution, which was a limitation of SAE. PIM detects non-linear echoes from microbubbles[17]. Alternate pulses, 180° out of phase, are transmitted down each ultrasound line and the summed echoes from the pair are used to form one image line. Echoes from linear and non-linear sources can be separated since non-linear signals, such as those from microbubbles, summate whilst linear signals cancel.

In a study of the specificity of SAE, spectrums of benign and malignant focal liver lesions were assessed for SAE activity in the late phase of Levovist[18]. Metastases and hepatocellular carcinoma (HCC) showed no or very low SAE signals whilst significantly higher uptake was observed in haemangiomas and focal nodular hyperplasia (FNH) (see Figures 1 and 2).

Imaging in late-phase PIM (LP-PIM) has been shown to increase sensitivity in the detection of focal liver malignancies[19,20]. In 20 patients, with known liver malignancies, LP-PIM significantly improved subjective and objective conspicuity[19] (see Figure 3). The smallest lesions detected decreased significantly from a mean of 11.5 mm in conventional B-Mode imaging (CBM) to 3.14 mm in LP-PIM, which were consistently noted in all patients. Significantly more lesions were detected on LP-PIM than CBM in all cases and, in 3 cases, more than on dual-phase CT. Importantly, no patient was understaged on LP-PIM compared with CBM and CT. Other studies have also shown that imaging the late phase of Levovist in SAE and PIM helps to characterize splenic lesions[21,22] thereby increasing diagnostic confidence. Multicentre trials looking at characterization of liver lesions using ADI are underway.

DIFFUSE LIVER DISEASE

There is no satisfactory non-invasive test to assess diffuse liver disease apart from a liver biopsy. The development of micro arteriovenous shunting in the liver with fibrosis and cirrhosis and an increased vascular supply in malignancy is well known and can be studied using a bolus of microbubbles as a tracer. In practice, a hepatic vein is interrogated with spectral Doppler following an intravenous bolus of a microbubble (Levovist). The audio output from the ultrasound system is fed via an analogue to digital converter to a computer which records the mean spectral

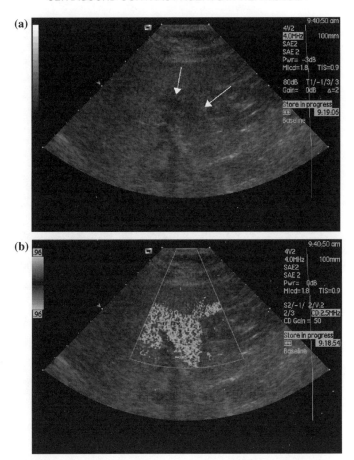

Figure 1 (a) Longitudinal section through the left lobe of the liver reveals an echo-poor lesion (arrows). (b) Three minutes after Levovist, imaging in SAE mode shows signal within the lesion consistent with benignity. Biopsy subsequently confirmed focal nodular hyperplasia (FNH). (Reproduced by kind permission of publishers Springer Verlag from 'Developments in ultrasound contrast media'. European Radiology 2001[1])

intensity over each second, allowing a time intensity curve to be derived. An exponential smoothing algorithm is applied to the curve and the arrival time of the bolus (defined as a 10% rise in intensity above baseline) can be calculated.

In normal subjects, the arrival time usually occurs after 40 s. However, in cirrhosis and malignancy, an early arrival time (<24 s) and a 'left shift' of the time intensity curve is found because of an increased hepatic arterial supply and arteriovenous shunting. This technique has been shown to be a highly sensitive indicator of cirrhosis and metastases[23,24]. A study comparing 15 patients with biopsy-proven cirrhosis, 12 with biopsy-proven non-cirrhotic diffuse liver disease and 11 normal controls showed that an arrival time of 24 s or less in a hepatic vein was extremely sensitive in separating cirrhotic patients from the other two groups[23]. Large prospective trials are presently underway to assess the predictive

MEDICAL IMAGING IN GASTROENTEROLOGY AND HEPATOLOGY

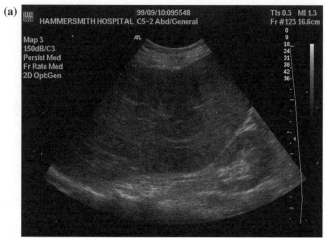

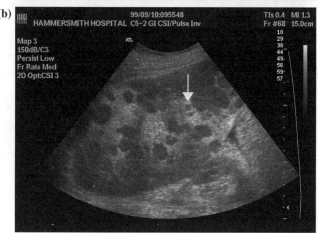

Figure 2 (a) Longitudinal section through the right lobe of liver in a patient with colorectal cancer. Conventional B-mode shows a heterogenous liver echo pattern but no definite focal lesions can be identified. (b) Five minutes after Levovist administration, insonation of the same area using phase inversion mode (PIM), reveals multiple metastases. Lesions as small as 3 mm can be identified (arrow). (Reproduced by kind permission of publishers Springer Verlag from 'Developments in ultrasound contrast media'. European Radiology 2001[1])

value of this technique in the development of metastases in cancer patients and as a non-invasive method of grading diffuse liver disease.

FUTURE APPLICATIONS OF MICROBUBBLES

Microbubbles may be used as vehicles for the delivery of therapeutic agents[25]. These could include delivery of genes, thrombolytics and oncological drugs specifically to the liver for maximal efficacy.

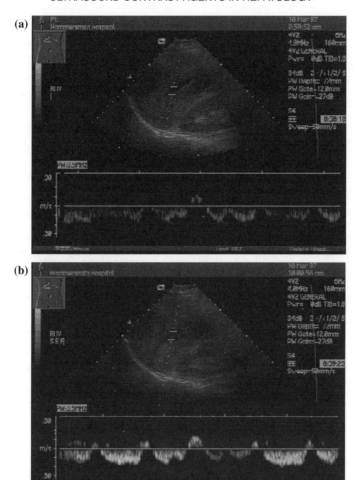

Figure 3 (a) Spectral Doppler study of a right hepatic vein pre-administration of Levovist. (b) Following Levovist, there is marked enhancement of the Doppler signal. The time from injection to the enhancement effect can be measured and can provide an index for diffuse liver disease (see text). (Reproduced by kind permission of publishers Springer Verlag from 'Developments in ultrasound contrast media'. European Radiology 2001[1])

SUMMARY

Microbubble contrast agents have markedly extended the clinical and research applications of ultrasound. They allow better liver lesion characterization and, with tissue-specific agents, improved detection of focal liver lesions to rival that of CT and MR. Functional studies are promising for assessing diffuse liver disease and exciting applications for the role of microbubbles in therapeutics are being developed.

References

1. Harvey CJ, Blomley MJK, Eckersley RJ, Cosgrove DO. Developments in ultrasound contrast media. Eur Radiol. 2001;11:675–89.
2. Goldberg BB. Ultrasound contrast agents, 2nd edn. London: Martin Dunitz, 2001.
3. Nanda N, Carstensen EL. Echo-enhancing agents: safety. In: Nanda N, Schlief R, Goldberg BB, editions. Advances in Echo Imaging Using Contrast Enhancement. 2nd edn. Lancaster, England: Kluwer Academic, 1997:115–31.
4. Schlief R. Developments in echo-enhancing agents. Clin Rad. 1996;51(Suppl 1):5–7.
5. Schneider M, Arditi M, Barrau MB et al. BR1: a new ultrasonographic contrast agent based on sulphur hexachloride-filled microbubbles. Invest Radiol. 1995;30:451–7.
6. Bauer A, Mahler M, Urbank A, Zomack M, Schlief R, Niendorf HP. Microvascular imaging: results from a phase 1 study of the novel polymeric contrast agent SHU 563A. In: Nanda N, Schlief R, Goldberg BB, eds. Advances in Echo Imaging Using Contrast Enhancement, 2nd edn. Lancaster, England: Kluwer Academic, 1997:685–90.
7. Eckersley RJ, Cosgrove DO, Blomley MJ, Hashimoto H. Functional imaging of tissue response to bolus injection of ultrasound contrast agent. In: Proceedings of the IEEE Ultrasonics Symposium 2. 1998:1779–82.
8. Walker KW, Pantely GA, Sahn DJ. Ultrasound mediated destruction of contrast agents: effects of ultrasound intensity, exposure and frequency. Invest Radiol. 1997;32:728–34.
9. Choi D, Lim HK, Kim SH et al. Hepatocellular carcinoma treated with percutaneous radiofrequency ablation: usefulness of power Doppler US with a microbubble contrast agent in evaluating therapeutic response-preliminary results. Radiology. 2000;217:558–63.
10. Clement O, Siauve N, Cuenod C-A, Frija G. Liver imaging with ferumoxides (feridex): fundamentals, controversies and practical aspects. Topics Magn Resonance Imag. 1998; 9:167–82.
11. Albrecht T, Blomley MJK, Heckemann RA et al. Stimulated acoustic emission with the US contrast agent Levovist: a clinically useful contrast effect with liver-specific properties. RöFo Fortschr Geb Rontgenstr Neuen Bildgeb Verfahr. 2000;172:61–7.
12. Blomley MJK, Albrecht T, Cosgrove DO et al. Stimulated acoustic emission in the liver parenchyma with the US contrast agent Levovist. Lancet. 1998;351:568.
13. Blomley MJK, Albrecht T, Cosgrove DO et al. Stimulated acoustic emission to image a late liver and spleen-specific phase of Levovist in normal volunteers and patients with and without liver disease. US Med Biol. 1999;25:1341–52.
14. Leen E, Ramnarine K, Kyriakopoulou, K et al. Improved characterization of focal liver tumors: Dynamic doppler imaging using NC100100: A new liver specific echo-enhancer. Eur J Ultrasound. 2000;11:95–104.
15. Schneider M, Broillet A, Bussat P et al. Gray-scale liver enhancement in VX2 tumor-bearing rabbits using BR14, a new ultrasonographic contrast agent. Invest Radiol. 1997;32:410–17.
16. Hauff P, Fritzsch T, Reinhardt M et al. Delineation of experimental liver tumors in rabbits by a new US contrast agent and stimulated acoustic emission. Invest Radiol. 1997;32:94–9.
17. Hope Simpson D, Chin CT, Burns PN. Pulse inversion Doppler: A new method for detecting non-linear echoes from microbubble contrast agents. IEEE Trans Ultrasonics Ferroelectrics Frequency Control. 1999;46:372–82.
18. Blomley MJK, Sidhu PS, Cosgrove DO et al. Do different types of liver lesions differ in their uptake of the microbubble SH U 508A in its late liver phase: Early experience. Radiology. 2001;220:661–7.
19. Heckemann RA, Cosgrove DO, Blomley MJ, Eckersley RJ, Harvey CJ, Mine Y. Liver lesions: intermittent second-harmonic grey-scale US can increase conspicuity with microbubble contrast material-early experience. Radiology. 2000;216:592–6.
20. Harvey CJ, Blomley MJK, Eckersley RJ, Heckemann RA, Butler-Barnes J, Cosgrove DO. Pulse inversion mode imaging of liver specific microbubbles: Improved detection of subcentimetre metastases. Lancet. 2000;355:870–08.
21. Forsberg F, Goldberg BB, Liu JB et al. Tissue-specific US contrast agent for evaluation of hepatic and splenic parenchyma. Radiology. 1999;210:125–32.
22. Harvey CJ, Blomley MJK, Cosgrove DO, Eckersley RJ, Heckemann R, Butler-Barnes J. Characterisation of splenic lesions using pulse inversion mode and stimulated acoustic emission (SAE) imaging with the ultrasound contrast agent levovist. Eur Radiol. 1999;10(Suppl 1):S144.

23. Albrecht T, Blomley MJK, Cosgrove DO et al. Non-invasive diagnosis of hepatic cirrhosis by transit-time analysis of an ultrasound contrast agent. Lancet. 1999;353:1579–83.
24. Blomley MJK, Albrecht T, Cosgrove DO et al. Liver vascular transit time analyzed with dynamic hepatic venography with bolus injections of an US contrast agent: Early experience in 7 patients with metastases. Radiology. 1998;209:862–6.
25. Unger EC. Targeting and delivery of drugs with contrast agents. In: Thomsen HS, Muller RN, Mattrey RF (eds) Trends in Contrast Media. Medical Radiology: Diagnostic Imaging and Radiation Oncology Series. Berlin: Springer, 1999:405–12.

16
Percutaneous interventional therapy of liver cancer

T. LIVRAGHI

HEPATOCELLULAR CARCINOMA

Introduction

In countries where ultrasound (US) screening of a population at risk is practised, early diagnosis of hepatocellular carcinoma (HCC) is possible, whereas elsewhere, apart from the odd incidental finding, the diagnosis is not made until the disease is already advanced. The time of diagnosis governs the type of treatment offered: possibly curative when diagnosis is early, palliative or nothing when diagnosis is late. The range of treatment options is fairly wide, and the choice is not always easy, given the number of variables to be assessed. The options open today are the following: surgical, interstitial (or percutaneous ablation techniques), intra-arterial, systemic and radiant. Most of these have not been validated with randomized controlled studies, i.e. versus the natural history or versus other therapies, but are applied only on the basis of the local control of the tumour. The impact on survival of most interventions was measured against historical data. Therefore selection bias cannot altogether be ruled out.

The survival studies of untreated patients usually taken as points of reference fall into three conventional and gross groups: those relating to patients in whom the disease was at an early stage (single HCC < 5 cm, or up to three lesions <3 cm) and therefore likely to be amenable to curative treatment; those in whom the disease was considered intermediate, i.e. all the other stages without an invasive tumour pattern (absence of portal thrombosis or extrahepatic spread) and not allowing symptoms; and those in whom the disease was considered advanced or terminal.

The first group includes patients recruited retrospectively who have not been treated for several reasons. Their 3-year survival ranges between 13% and 21%[1,2], reaching 30% in 47 Child class A patients with a single HCC < 5 cm and deemed potentially operable. The figures were obtained years ago when imaging examinations were less accurate, so an understaging was probable. However, in the future it will be very difficult to carry out a prospective trial considering such patients for ethical reasons, the current availability of no-risk therapeutic options, and the migration of patients. In confirmation of the poor confidence of the aforementioned studies, a clearly higher survival rate in patients (prospectively recruited) with an intermediate stage was recently reported[3]. Their 1-, 3-, and 5-year survival was 80%, 50% and 16%, respectively, with a median survival of 40 months. Such a study, which needs confirmation in additional trials, opened a debate, since it questioned the previous results of several series of established invasive therapies, such as partial resection or conventional transarterial chemoembolization (TACE). In fact, the survival of the treated patients was frequently shorter than that of the aforementioned untreated patients, even though with a more adverse profile. A national study based in Japan demonstrated 1-year, 3-year and 5-year survival of 67%, 40% and 29%, respectively, in 2174 consecutively resected cases[4]. The explanation could be that selection was not strict, or that some potential severe side-effects worsened the natural course of the disease.

Before going into the various aspects of the therapeutic choice, three fundamental premises for the evaluation and hence management of the patient need to be stated. The first premise concerns the coexisting chronic liver disease, the second the multifocal origin of HCC, and the third the factors affecting prognosis.

The underlying chronic hepatic disease, generally of viral origin (primarily hepatitis C infection), accompanies the neoplastic disease in different stages of its course. According to the stage, one disease will prevail over the other. Usually a patient with chronic hepatitis will die of the tumour, whereas a patient with advanced cirrhosis will die of liver failure. For such reasons therapies should not worsen liver function.

It is known, though only confirmed a few years ago, that HCC should be considered an organ disease, since it has been proven to be multicentric in origin. The implication of the fact, which should always be borne in mind in patient management, is that the only treatment likely to afford permanent cure is orthotopic liver transplantation (OLT). Most resected patients present new lesions in other segments at 5 years of follow-up. The factor associated with the highest new recurrences rate stemmed from an active inflammation.

The search for predictive factors has led, through more far-reaching knowledge of the disease, to more appropriate patient management. Better assessment has made a more accurate selection possible, thereby safeguarding patients from useless or even harmful interventions. It is understood that such factors may vary depending on the type of treatment. For example, whereas portal thrombosis is always deleterious irrespective of the treatment, increasing size is an adverse factor more for percutaneous ablation techniques than for resection. Clearly, there cannot always be rigid criteria for exclusion of a given treatment on the grounds of one or more adverse factors, if the patient stands to benefit from it. However, the greater the risk for the patient, the more careful selection should be, especially if alternative therapies carrying less risk and lower cost are available. The best-known adverse prognostic factors have been validated by means of statistical analysis, even though the results are sometimes discordant. They are: vascular invasion, high alpha-fetoprotein, satellites, low grade, abnormal bilirubin, portal hypertension, high transaminases, non-anatomical resection, too advanced age, Child B class, or multifocality[4–9]. Other prognostic factors, such as oestrogen receptors, are emerging[10].

Before evaluating the role of percutaneous techniques, other therapies applicable to the same type of patients (i.e. with early or intermediate HCC) need to be considered.

OLT

The procedure is the sole treatment able to remove the still-unknown preneoplastic nodules together with the tumour itself as well as the coexistent chronic liver disease, which can only deteriorate. The Paris Consensus Conference of 1994 produced the following guidelines: any type of extrahepatic spread is a contraindication to OLT, an unresectable tumour at UICC stage II is a favourable indication, and a UICC stage III or IV tumour is a borderline individual decision[11]. However, the selection criteria at the leading centres are somewhat discordant. For instance, starting from the assumption that partial resection can be only a palliative option, the King's College London team considers OLT the treatment of choice for Child's classes B and C with a single HCC < 8 cm and, given the high incidence of satellites and multifocal lesions found in explanted liver but not diagnosed by imaging in the work-up for OLT, probably also for Child's class A[12] with single HCC < 8 cm. In any case, resorting to OLT is limited severely by the availability of donors, so that most centres prefer to perform OLT following the cut-off of Milan criteria, confirmed by other studies, i.e. only when the tumour is at early stage, because of the excellent results obtained (5-year survival of 75%) with a very low recurrence rate[13,14]. However, the shortage of donors has also resulted in an increase in waiting time, thereby allowing the tumour to grow to stages that may contraindicate the intervention. When the waiting time exceeds 6 months, 23–50% of patients are excluded from OLT. The event greatly worsens patient outcome when assessing the OLT results according to intention-to-treat[15]. In summary, OLT unfortunately remains a chimaeric option for most patients, since demand largely exceeds supply (in Italy alone the number of new cases of HCC is estimated at around 10 000 a year, whereas the number of OLT performed in a year is less than 100), since high costs and advanced technology preclude it in poorer countries where HCC is more common, and since a highly developed country such as Japan refuses to adopt it for ethical reasons. To increase the number of OLT, some new strategies, such as split liver, marginal livers and liver from living donors, have recently been proposed.

Partial resection

In Western countries only about 10–15% of patients with HCC may receive resection, although its applicability seems higher in Eastern countries, probably due to the wider and closer use of ultrasound screening. The indications range from an ideal situation – that is, one in which the patient <65 years is Child's class A with a single encapsulated small HCC at an easily operated site – to cases in which resection has to be very extensive because of an HCC at any stage of local–regional disease requiring vascular reconstruction due to portal and inferior vena cava tumour thrombi and resection of intrahepatic metastases in both lobes. Resection is feasible in both situations, but the operative risk and long-term survival differ greatly when major adverse prognostic factors are present. In any case, even when the tumour is small, an important problem for surgeons is what type of resection should be performed. The intervention can remove only the tumour (enucleation), the tumour with a safety margin of liver tissue around (wedge resection), or the tumour with the portal feeding area (anatomical resection). The extension of the latter resection ranges from the segment (segmentectomy), a part of it (sub-segmentectomy), or two adjacent segments on the basis of the order of the portal branch which is divided (bi-segmentectomy). The choices are dependent on liver function and surgical skill. Only anatomical resections can ensure the removal of satellites or microportal invasion not yet visible, and obtain longer survival[7].

In 1838 patients collected from 15 series with a single HCC <5 cm and well-compensated cirrhosis, the 5-year survival rates ranged from 33% to 64% with a mean of 51%, perioperative mortality from 1.4% to 11% with a mean of 7%, and a complication rate of up to 58%[16]. More recent series from leading centres report higher survival. Lau et al. obtained a 5-year survival of 72% in stage I and 55% in stage II, according to UICC staging[17]. The Liver Unit of Barcelona obtained a 5-year survival of 74% in strictly selected candidates, but only 25% in the worst candidates[5], i.e. those with portal hypertension and bilirubin >1 mg/dl. Perioperative mortality is also decreasing, reaching 0% in some of the leading centres but maintaining too high a level (13%) in others[18–20].

In summary, partial resection almost invariably achieves complete ablation (also of peripheral satellites if anatomical resection is carried out), but presents the following weak points: multifocality of the tumour in due time so that most patients die of HCC, underlying hepatic disease which can only progress, low operability rate and perioperative risk in asymptomatic patients with a good life expectation, loss of non-neoplastic tissue that in some interventions could hasten liver failure, and now the availability of competitive therapies.

Arterial (chemo) embolization

For many years transarterial embolization (TAE) or TACE of the whole liver was the most widely used option for patients with intermediate HCC. The rationale of the approach evolved from the fact that, in contrast to liver tissue, HCC receives almost all of its blood supply through the hepatic artery. TAE or TACE have been confirmed to have a marked anti-tumoral effect, even though only in encapsulated lesions. Surprisingly, three recent controlled randomized trials did not show any statistically significant difference in survival between treated and untreated patients[21–23]. Treated patients presented a slower tumour progression and even a decrease in the incidence of portal invasion, but the probability of presenting cancer-related complications or liver decompensation was not modified when compared to untreated patients. This is probably due to a counterbalance between local tumour control and damage to non-neoplastic tissue, which hastens liver insufficiency. In the recent study by the Liver Unit of Barcelona, 2- and 4-year survival was 49% and 13% after TAE and 50% and 27% after no treatment[22]. Perhaps further large randomized trials are still needed to clarify whether differences in the selection of patients may result in a therapeutic benefit for at least a subgroup of patients. Currently, the trend is to use TAE or TACE in patients inoperable or not treatable with percutaneous ablation procedures and to perform the lobar or only the segmental technique, which causes less deterioration in liver function than the whole-liver technique, while obtaining a better tumour response. Segmental or selected TACE has broadly the same indications as segmental resection or percutaneous interstitial techniques. As the treatment is confined to one segment or less, it presents no short-term complications or the problems of long-term liver function deterioration that mark the conventional intra-arterial approach. The 5-year survival among 173 patients collected from two series with HCC <5 cm, and whose cirrhosis was not advanced, ranged from 33% to 53%, with a mean of 44%[16]. In comparison, among 640 patients from five series with the same disease presentation, and treated with the conventional whole-liver approach, 5-year survival ranged from 9% to 32%, with a mean of 13%[16].

Percutaneous ablation techniques

The range of indications for interstitial treatments is becoming wider than for surgery and intra-arterial therapies. Indeed, whereas for some years only patients with up to three small (3 or <5 cm) lesions were treated, and this still applies at many centres, with the introduction of the 'single-session' procedures under general anaesthesia[24], even patients with lesions greater in number or larger in size are now being treated.

The following points constitute the rationale on which interstitial procedures are based: (a) percutaneous ethanol injection (PEI) or radio frequency (RF) do not have the disadvantage of loss or important damage of non-neoplastic parenchyma, in contrast with multisegmental resection or whole (lobar?)-liver TACE; (b) PEI and RF are low-risk procedures. In published series the mortality rate is insignificant (0.09% in the largest study of PEI)[25]; (c) PEI and RF can be easily repeated when new lesions appear, as happens in most patients within 5 years. Since new lesions reflect the natural history of the disease the patient should be followed frequently so that the new lesions can be treated as they form. An advantage is that the patient can be followed by the same physician in the diagnostic as well therapeutic phase; (d) the low cost, easy availability of the necessary material (particularly as regards PEI), and the simplicity of the techniques make it possible to perform them anywhere, even in peripheral centres. The patients are generally treated on an outpatient basis, and most of them can carry out normal daily life. In Italy the cost of one PEI cycle is about $1000, partial resection about $30 000 and OLT about $125 000. In Japan an average cost of $759 for outpatient PEI and $27 105 for resection was reported[16]. Since every year the number of patients who develop the disease is about 25 000 in Japan and 12 000 in Italy, the problem of costs is not of secondary importance.

An open question remains the choice between PEI and other ablation procedures. None of these has changed the rationale on which treatment PEI is based. From them we await only an increased percentage of complete necrosis while maintaining the safety of PEI.

There are only three comparative studies: one with acetic acid and two with RF. The first trial (randomized) reported better results, in terms of local efficacy, recurrence rate and survival, in favour of acetic acid[26]. However, the weak point of the study was that it was carried out by the inventor of the technique; surprisingly, his survival of patients treated with PEI was much lower than all the survivals reported by several other authors. Currently, no other studies have confirmed the aforementioned initial experience.

Both the trials (randomized) comparing RF and PEI in the treatment of small (<3 cm) HCC obtained better results in terms of local efficacy, local recurrence and treatment duration in favour of RF, the only advantage in favour of PEI being a lower rate of complications[27,28]. However, both the trials confirmed the efficacy of PEI and this means that PEI remains a valid tool where RF is not available.

In our department we use both techniques (and also segmental TACE), according to the features of the disease, i.e. size, number, location, margins, presence of satellites or portal thrombosis, and the response. A multifocal HCC can be treated with only one or with all the techniques, during a single hospital stay or over a period of years. For instance, in a patient with four lesions, three nodules can be treated with 'single-session' RF (or PEI) and the fourth with segmental TACE if it is located in the upper part of segment 8 and not recognizable at US examination. The same lesion can also be treated with the combination of different techniques. Most lesions are treated with RF ablation. RF obtains a higher rate of necrosis in small tumours (particularly in infiltrating lesions of any size) and avoids the side-effects occurring after single-session PEI when a large amount (>60 ml) of ethanol is required[29]; PEI is preferable in lesions at risk with RF, i.e. adjacent to main biliary ducts or to intestinal loops (above all when fibrotic adhesions between the hepatic capsule and intestinal wall are suspected), in lesions difficult to approach or protruding from the capsule, and when portal thrombosis is treatable[30]. Segmental TACE is used in lesions not recognizable at US examination, in lesions not completely necrotized and presenting the remnant vital tissue scattered or not recognizable at US examination for an additional treatment with RF or PEI, and in the presence of satellites after the achievement of complete necrosis of the main lesion.

Conclusions

The large number of patients enrolled in US screening programmes has created a demand for effective, safe, repeatable and economic treatment that can be made available in many centres. In the absence of randomized trials it is and will be very difficult to find a consensual agreement on the indications of the respective therapeutic options. In my opinion the only course at this time is to extrapolate from retrospective comparative studies, and from studies on prognostic factors, at least the unequivocal information that can prevent useless or even damaging therapies. Moreover, economic resources and the expertise available at each centre are other factors that have a certain role in the choice of treatment.

Although it is understood that partial resection assures the highest possibility to completely ablate the tumour, the survival rates after surgery are roughly comparable with those obtained with PEI[16,31]. The explanation is probably due to a balance among advantages and disadvantages of the two therapies. Moreover, the results of surgery have been hampered by incorrect selection of patients, part of them being resected even though carriers of adverse prognostic factors. PEI survival curves are always better than curves of resected patients who present adverse prognostic factors. Another confirmation of such an interpretation comes from the last report of the Liver Cancer Study Group of Japan[32]. Three- and 5-year survival in Child's class A patients with single HCC <5 cm was respectively 67% and 49% in the previous report of 1982–89 (when PEI was not available) and 77% and 59% in the last report of 1988–95 (75% and 46% with PEI) because of better patient selection (perioperative mortality remained substantially unchanged) and the probable shift to PEI of some patients who, before the advent of PEI, would have been treated surgically.

On the basis of the aforementioned studies, PEI or even better RF ablation (long-term results are not yet available but our initial results, i.e. 85% at the 3-year follow-up in single HCC <5 cm, anticipate an additional increase in the survival achieved with PEI) is indicated as the treatment of choice for most patients enrolled by US screening, excluding those candidate for OLT and for partial resection. Unfortunately, OLT is available for very few patients. Candidates for partial resection should present all the following factors:

1. (clinical) Child's class A, transaminases <3 times normal values, not too advanced an age, no portal hypertension, normal serum bilirubin;
2. (technical) perioperative mortality <3%, (sub)segmentectomy feasible;
3. (neoplastic) no portal thrombosis, AFP <600, single tumour (also with peripheral satellites, if anatomical resection is feasible).

However, it is still debated whether a complex resection is an appropriate choice for a patient without adverse prognostic factors and a small tumour, when the possibility of peritumoral microinvasion is low and the rate of complete ablation with percutaneous ablation techniques is almost 100%.

In practice, most patients could be managed as follows: early detection of the HCC by means of US screening in an at-risk population, treatment with PEI or RF, follow-up with imaging methods and tumour markers (AFP, DCP), and treatment of new lesions again with PEI or RF.

LIVER METASTASES

Partial resection

Only in the past few years was it (indirectly) demonstrated that surgical resection can radically cure some patients with liver metastases of colorectal origin. The statement was possible owing to the availability of very long-term survival curves that demonstrated patients free of disease after 10 years from the resection. No controlled randomized trials have been performed to compare treated and untreated patients, and the survivals of resected patients were generally compared with few and old studies on the natural history of patients not comparable and with more advanced disease. In untreated patients the longest survival reported was 23% and 8%, respectively, at the 3- and 5-year follow-up[33]. Two studies established the possible definitive cure[34,35]. In the first study the 5-year survival of resected patients was 27%, in line with several other survival curves ranging from 16% to 35%, but 10-year survival remained almost unchanged, i.e. 20%, with all patients free of disease. Only 7% of patients free of disease at the

5-year follow-up had recurrent tumour. The aforementioned study is also paradigmatic in relation to the history of resected patients. In total, 280 patients were treated with a potentially curative aim. All detectable tumour was completely removed at the time of the operation. Overall survival for all patients was 84% at 1 year, 46% at 3 years, and 27% at 5 years. Median survival was 2.7 years. Recurrent disease was the cause of death in 83% of the entire series. Perioperative mortality was 4% at 60 days. In the study by Fong et al.[35] 5- and 10-year survival was 37% and 22%, respectively, and perioperative mortality was 2.8%.

In practice, historical evidence shows that only one-third of patients with liver metastases from colorectal cancer are candidate for resection, and such studies show that 20–22% of the one-third will be definitely cured, i.e. 6–7% of the total population.

Is it possible to select the patients who will potentially have a definitive cure? There are different points of view on this problem.

Most centres currently select the patient according to some prognostic factors. The most relevant study concerning the enrollment of patients following such a trend was recently carried out by Fong and co-workers[35]. Seven factors were identified to be significant and independent predictors of poor long-term outcome by multivariate analysis: positive margin, extrahepatic disease, node-positive primary, disease-free interval from primary to metastases <12 months, number of hepatic tumours >1, largest hepatic tumour >5 cm, and CEA level >200 ng/ml. When the last five of the criteria were used in a preoperative scoring system, assigning one point for each criterion, the total score was highly predictive of outcome ($p < 0.0001$). No patient with a score of 5 was a long-term survivor. The authors concluded that patients with up to two criteria can have even a favourable outcome, whereas the others should be considered for experimental adjuvant trials.

A more aggressive approach considers as selection criteria only the possibility of an oncologically radical operation and the possibility to preserve at least 40% of the normal tissue[36]. Using such an approach, even though the presence of some prognostic factors (stage of primary, lymph node metastases, multiple nodules, short interval between primary and metastatic tumour, and high level of CEA) was significantly associated with a poor prognosis, the authors obtained an overall 3-, 5-, and 10-year survival of 51%, 38%, and 26%, respectively, with zero perioperative mortality.

An interesting policy recommended by some researchers is the application of 'a test of time'[37,38]. They believe that the survival benefit from hepatic resection is determined by the biological features of the tumour rather than by early detection, and theorize that, by delaying intervention for 3–6 months, occult metastases will become evident. In this way patients who would not be cured by resection are identified and spared non-curative exploration or resection. A recent study[39] supported such a policy. In this experience, survival of patients who underwent resection for synchronous lesions after interval re-evaluation was significantly better than that of patients who underwent immediate resection, i.e. 5-year survival of 45% vs 7%, respectively, and in the meantime 64% of the re-evaluated patients was spared the morbidity of laparotomy. Also for patients with metachronous metastases who underwent interval re-evaluation, 29% was spared the morbidity of laparotomy because of an increased number of hepatic or distant metastases, whereas survival rates were not significantly better.

Percutaneous ablation techniques

What is the place of percutaneous interstitial techniques?

PEI was abandoned, except for endocrine lesions, when thermal procedures were proposed, since its efficacy was not as satisfying as with HCC. Although thermal ablation procedures present relevant advantages over surgery, such as minimal invasiveness with a 0% mortality rate and significantly lower complications, reduced costs and hospital stay, resection remains the gold standard because it is almost always able to assure complete ablation. Very recently, Vogl et al.[40] presented the first 5-year survival details of patients with colorectal metastases treated with a thermal technique, and the rate was 30%. It is noteworthy that the most of the patients were considered inoperable, so that a better survival might be expected in comparable operable patients. However, ablation techniques are size- and site-dependent and are not always able to assure a complete necrosis also in lesions <3 cm.

Of course, other liver metastases from different primaries have been treated, but since the subgroups were too limited in number it is currently difficult to reach any conclusion. However, from our personal experience with RF we have learned that the volume of necrosis can change according to the histotype, because of the differences in tissue conduction and vascularization.

Only a group of patients with breast metastases presented a number sufficiently consistent to reach a conclusion[41]. Twenty-four patients with 64 lesions were treated, and complete necrosis was obtained in 92% of them. Ten of 16 patients with lesions initially confined to the liver were free of disease during a follow-up ranging from 4 to 44 months. The authors concluded that, even though the proportion of patients with liver-only metastases (or maybe also with stable bone disease) was relatively low, the high overall prevalence of breast cancer suggested that a certain number of patients may be eligible for RF treatment.

CONCLUSIONS

Partial resection is the first choice among local treatments. Percutaneous thermal procedures are indicated in patients who are unresectable or who refuse surgery. However, on the basis of the studies on 'test of time', a possible candidate could be a patient presenting synchronous (and maybe metachronous) operable metastases with favourable criteria (small size, accessible site) for a complete ablation. In such a case the follow-up could offer the following possibilities, according to the response and the natural course of the disease: (a) the lesion treated is completely ablated; whether new lesions appear or not, the patient has avoided surgery; (b) the treated lesion presents partial necrosis or local recurrence. If no new lesions appear the patient can be resected, whereas if new lesions appear the patient is spared a useless operation.

Systemic chemotherapy or intra-arterial hepatic chemotherapy can be used according to the local policy.

References

1. Ebara M, Ohto M, Shinagawa T et al. Natural history of minute hepatocellular carcinoma smaller than three centimeters complicating cirrhosis. A study in 22 patients. Gastroenterology. 1986;90:289–98.

2. Livraghi T, Bolondi L, Buscarini L et al. No treatment, resection and ethanol injection in hepatocellular carcinoma: a retrospective analysis of survival in 391 patients with cirrhosis. J Hepatol. 1995;22:522–6.
3. Llovet JM, Bru C, Bruix J. Prognosis of hepatocellular carcinoma: the BCLC staging classification. Semin Liver Dis. 1999;19:329–39.
4. Liver Cancer Study Group of Japan. Predictive factors for long term prognosis after partial hepatectomy for patients with hepatocellular carcinoma in Japan. Cancer. 1994;74:2772–80.
5. Bruix J, Castells A, Bosch J et al. Surgical resection of hepatocellular carcinoma in cirrhotic patients: prognosis value of preoperative portal pressure. Gastroenterology. 1996;3:1018–22.
6. Noun R, Jagot P, Farges O, Sauvanet A, Belghiti J. High preoperative serum alanine transferase levels: effect on the risk of liver resection in Child grade A cirrhotic patients. World J Surg. 1997;21:390–5.
7. Takayama T, Makuuchi M. Surgical resection. In: Livraghi T, Makuuchi M, Buscarini L, eds. Diagnosis and Treatment of Hepatocellular Carcinoma. London: Greenwich Medical Media, 1997:279–94.
8. Fong Y, Sun RL, Jarnagin W, Blumgart LH. An analysis of 412 cases of hepatocellular carcinoma at a western center. Ann Surg. 1999;229:790–800.
9. Poon RTP, Fan ST, Lo CM, Liu CL, Ng IOL, Wong J. Long-term prognosis after resection of hepatocellular carcinoma associated with hepatitis B-related cirrhosis. J Clin Oncol. 2000;18:1094–101.
10. Villa E, Moles A, Ferretti I et al. Natural history of inoperable hepatocellular carcinoma: estrogen receptors' status in the tumor is the strongest prognostic factor for survival. Hepatology. 2000;32:233–8.
11. Consensus statement on indications for liver transplantation: Paris, 22–23 June, 1993. Hepatology. 1994;20:635–85.
12. Tan KC, Rela M, Ryder SD et al. Experience of orthotopic liver transplantation and hepatic resection for hepatocellular carcinoma of less than 8 cm in patients with cirrhosis. Br J Surg. 1995;82:253–6.
13. Mazzaferro V, Regalia E, Doci R, Andreola S, Pulvirenti A. Liver transplantation for treatment of small hepatocellular carcinomas in patients with cirrhosis. N Engl J Med. 1996;334:693–9.
14. Bismuth H, Majno PE, Adam R. Liver transplantation for hepatocellular carcinoma. Semin Liver Dis. 1999;19:311–22.
15. Llovet JM, Fuster J, Bruix J. Intention-to-treat analysis of surgical treatment for early hepatocellular carcinoma: resection versus transplantation. Hepatology. 1999;30:1434–40.
16. Livraghi T, Giorgio A, Marin G et al. Hepatocellular carcinoma and cirrhosis in 746 patients: long-term results of percutaneous ethanol injection. Radiology. 1995;197:101–8.
17. Lau H, Tat Fan S, Ng I et al. Long term prognosis after hepatectomy for hepatocellular carcinoma. Cancer. 1998;83:2302–11.
18. Fan TS, Lo C, Liu C. Hepatectomy for hepatocellular carcinoma: toward zero hospital deaths. Ann Surg. 1999;229:322–30.
19. Torzilli G, Makuuchi M, Inoue K et al. No-mortality liver resection for hepatocellular carcinoma in cirrhotic and noncirrhotic patients. Arch Surg. 1999;134:984–92.
20. Paquet KJ, Gad HA, Lazar A et al. Analysis of factors affecting outcome after hepatectomy of patients with liver cirrhosis and small hepatocellular carcinoma. Eur J Surg. 1998;164:513–19.
21. Group d'Etude et de Traitement de Carcinome Hepatocellulaire. A comparison of lipiodol chemoembolization and conservative treatment for unresectable hepatocellular carcinoma. N Engl J Med. 1995;332:1256–61.
22. Bruix J, Llovet JM, Castells A et al. Transarterial embolization versus symptomatic treatment in patients with advanced hepatocellular carcinoma. Results of a randomized controlled trial in a single institution. Hepatology. 1998;27:1578–83.
23. Pelletier G, Ducreux M, Gay F et al. Treatment of unresectable hepatocellular carcinoma with lipiodol chemoembolization: a multicenter randomized trial. J Hepatol. 1998;29:129–34.
24. Livraghi T, Vettori C, Torzilli G, Lazzaroni S, Pellicanò S, Ravasi S. Percutaneous ethanol injection of hepatic tumors: single session therapy under general anesthesia. Am J Roentgenol. 1993;160:1065–9.
25. Di Stasi M, Buscarini L, Livraghi T et al. Percutaneous ethanol injection in the treatment of hepatocellular carcinoma: a multicenter survey of evaluation practices and complications rates. Scand J Gastroenterol. 1997;32:1168–73.

26. Ohnishi K, Yoshioka H, Ito S, Fujiwara K. Prospective randomized controlled trial comparing percutaneous acetic acid injection and percutaneous ethanol injection for small hepatocellular carcinoma. Hepatology. 1998;27:67–72.
27. Livraghi T, Goldberg N, Lazzaroni S, Meloni F, Solbiati L, Gazelle S. Small hepatocellular carcinoma: treatment with radio-frequency ablation versus ethanol injection. Radiology. 1999;210:655–61.
28. Lencioni R, Cioni D, Donati F, Crocetti L, Granai G, Bartolozzi L. Percutaneous treatment of small hepatocellular carcinoma in cirrhosis: RF thermal ablation vs PEI. A prospective randomized trial. Radiology. 1999;213(P):123.
29. Livraghi T, Benedini V, Lazzaroni S, Meloni F, Torzilli G, Vettori C. Long term results of single session PEI in patients with large hepatocellular carcinoma. Cancer. 1998;83:48–57.
30. Livraghi T, Grigioni W, Mazziotti A, Sangalli G, Vettori C. Percutaneous ethanol injection of portal thrombosis in hepatocellular carcinoma: a new possible treatment. Tumori. 1990;76: 394–7.
31. Ryu M, Shimamura Y, Kinoshita T et al. Therapeutic results of resection, TAE and PEI in 3225 patients with hepatocellular. Jpn J Clin Oncol. 1997;27:251–7.
32. Liver Cancer Study Group of Japan. Survey and follow-up of primary cancer in Japan: report 12: Acta Hepatol Jpn. 1997;38:35–48.
33. Wagner JS, Adson MA, Van Heerden JA et al. The natural history of hepatic metastases from colorectal cancer: a comparison with resective treatment. Ann Surg. 1984;199:502–8.
34. Jamison RL, Donohue JH, Nagorney DM, Rosen CB, Harmsen WS, Ilsrtup DM. Hepatic resection for metastatic colorectal cancer results in cure for some patients. Arch Surg. 1997;132:505–11.
35. Fong Y, Forter J, Sun RL, Brennan MF, Blumgart LH. Clinical score for predicting recurrence after hepatic resection for metastatic colorectal cancer. Ann Surg. 1999;230:309–21.
36. Minagawa M, Makuuchi M, Torzilli G et al. Extension of the frontiers of surgical indications in the treatment of liver metastases from colorectal cancer. Ann Surg. 2000;231:487–99.
37. Cady B, Stone L. The role of surgical resection of liver metastases in colorectal carcinoma. Semin Oncol. 1991;18:399–406.
38. Scheele J. Hepatectomy for liver metastases. Br J Surg. 1993;80:274–6.
39. Lambert LA, Colacchio TA, Barth RJ. Interval hepatic resection of colorectal metastases improves patient selection. Arch Surg. 2000;135:473–80.
40. Vogl TJ, Mack MG, Schmitt J, Engelmann KS, Zangos S, Straub R. Can MR-guided LITT replace surgery in colorectal liver metastases?. Radiology. 2000;217(P):538.
41. Livraghi T, Meloni F, Goldberg SN, Gazelle GS, Lazzaroni S, Solbiati L. Radiofrequency (RF) ablation for the treatment of breast cancer liver metastases. Radiology. 2001;220:145–9.

17
Clinical role of ultrasound in biliary disease

S. WAGNER

INTRODUCTION

Ultrasound is the least invasive radiological modality for imaging the liver and biliary tract. Unlike CT scanning and magnetic resonance imaging (MRI), ultrasound is very cost-effective, rapidly available and portable. In addition, it can be used to guide interventional procedures. Therefore, ultrasound remains the primary screening procedure for evaluation of the hepatobiliary system[1-6]. Ultrasound uses no ionizing radiation to create the image, and is therefore also the technique of choice in pregnant women, in patients with contrast allergies, or in those in whom MRI is contraindicated.

ULTRASOUND DIRECTS MANAGEMENT OF JAUNDICE

Ultrasound plays a central role in the management of patients with jaundice. Following history, physical examination, and determination of basic laboratory tests, ultrasound enables the physician to distinguish between obstructive jaundice and cholestatic liver disease (Figure 1). Ultrasound not only allows the detection of obstructive jaundice but may also define the cause and the level of obstruction with a sensitivity and specificity varying between 55–91% and 82–95%, respectively[7,8]. A recent study by Harvey & Miller has shown that initial ultrasound is better than initial CT in patients suspected of having acute biliary disease[9]. Follow-up CT within 48 h did not provide additional information regarding the biliary system. Therefore, its use should be limited to those patients with a wider differential diagnosis or with confusing clinical symptoms and signs.

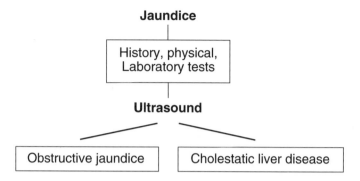

Figure 1 The role of ultrasound in the evaluation of jaundice

SPECIFIC ROLE OF ULTRASOUND IN BILIARY DISEASE

Gallbladder pathology

Cholecystolithiasis

Ultrasound is the gold standard for the diagnosis of cholecystolithiasis. Sonographic criteria of gallstones include polymorphic, hyperechoic reflections with or without shadowing (Figure 2). Gallstones are mostly position dependent. Cholesterol-pigment-lime stones represent 80% of gallstones and are sonolucent, whereas cholesterol stones are large and floating. Bilirubin stones are rare and are a sign of infection. The sensitivity and specificity of ultrasound for detection of gallstones >2 mm are higher than 95%[6]. CT scanning is not as accurate for detecting gallbladder wall abnormalities of gallstones; cholesterol stones can have the same density as bile.

Choledocholithiasis

Ultrasound has similar sensitivity to CT for detecting choledocholithiasis. The sensitivity of ultrasound for direct detection of common bile duct (CBD) stones amounts to 50%, whereas sensitivity rises to 75% if CBD is dilated >6 mm. Therefore, conventional ultrasound can only confirm, but not exclude, CBD stones. However, the diagnostic value of endoscopic ultrasound (EUS) is similar to that of cholangiography[10] (Figure 3). The sensitivity of EUS for detection of bile duct stones is 93%, specificity 97%, positive predictive value (PPV) 98%, and negative predictive value (NPV) 88%, respectively. Thus EUS can be used in lieu of ERCP for excluding CBD stones. If bile duct stones are suspected, ERCP

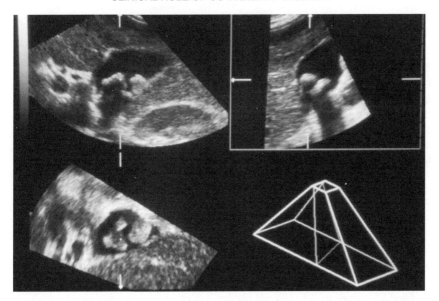

Figure 2 3D ultrasound of cholecystolithiasis. Cross, longitudinal and horizontal sections of the gallbladder are depicted

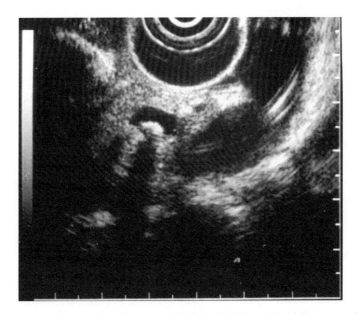

Figure 3 Endoscopic ultrasound of choledocholithiasis. Radial scanning of the common bile duct (7.5 MHz)

allows for detection and extraction of stones in a single session, and is therefore the method of choice in this situation.

Cholecystitis

Ultrasound plays a pre-eminent role in the diagnosis of cholecystitis[1,6]. An important ultrasound feature of cholecystitis is focal pain under direct pressure of the visualized gallbladder (Murphy's sign). This criterion has a positive predictive value of >90% for the diagnosis of cholecystitis. Further ultrasound criteria include wall thickening (diameter >4 mm), 3-layered wall, and a facultatively hypoechoic band around the gallbladder (pericholecystitis). Ultrasound is considered as the method of choice for diagnosis of cholecystitis and for evaluation of its complications. Typical complications comprise gallbladder hydrops (size >10 × 4 cm), perforation (covered, free), air in gallbladder (resulting from gas-forming bacteria or perforation), and empyema (hyperechoic lumen).

Gallbladder polyps

Three histological types of gallbladder polyps may by distinguished: (1) cholesterol polyps, (2) adenomyomatosis, and (3) neoplastic polyps. Sixty to 80% of gallbladder polyps are cholesterol polyps, which are non-neoplastic, 2–10 mm in size, and mostly multiple[11]. Cholesterol polyps are characterized by mucosal thickening, which is due to phagocytosis by histiocytes. Cholesterol polyps may be distinguished from cholesterol stones by power Doppler sonography through visualization of vessels inside the lesion. Adenomyomatosis is characterized by local thickening of the fundic wall (hourglass shape) and comprises 25% of gallbladder polyps. Adenomyomatosis is non-neoplastic, typically solitary with a size of 15 mm. Ademomas are neoplastic and encompass 4% of the gallbladder polyps. They coexist with gall stones in 50% of cases, their typical size range is between 5 and 20 mm, and they are solitary in about two thirds of cases. Ultrasound is the method of choice for the diagnosis and follow-up of gallbladder polyps. Cholecystectomy is indicated if the polyps are larger than 15 mm, grow in size more than 5 mm per year, and/or are symptomatic or demonstrate suspicious aspects.

Gallbladder cancer

Porcelain gallbladder is a premalign condition. Ultrasound criteria of porcelain gallbladder include hyperechoic, calcified wall, intramural deposits, semilunar shape, and shadowing. About 20% of such patients develop gallbladder cancer; therefore, prophylactic cholecystectomy is indicated. Ultrasound is the method of choice for diagnosis of porcelain gallbladder. Gallbladder cancer is sonographically characterized by polymorphic, irregular, hypoechoic changes in the gallbladder wall[12]. Two pathological types are differentiated: papillary and scirrhous carcinoma. Ultrasound is not suited to early diagnosis of gallbladder cancer. Endoscopic ultrasound may improve the sensitivity of the diagnosis of gallbladder cancer[13]. Loss of multiple-layer patterns of the gallbladder wall seems to be the most specific finding in diagnosing gallbladder cancer by endoscopic ultrasound.

Bile duct pathology

Infectious cholangitis

There are no direct criteria for diagnosis of infectious cholangitis by ultrasound[14]. Indirect evidence, such as dilated bile ducts and mucosal swelling, suggests the presence of acute cholangitis. Chronic cholangitis may present with bright reflexes of the wall, wall thickening, swelling of the mucosa within the CBD, and lymph nodes in the liver hilus. The diagnostic value of ultrasound is that of a screening method: i.e. detection of bile duct obstruction and dilatation. The gold standard for the diagnosis of cholangitis is ERCP for visualization of the bile ducts. In the near future, MRCP may become the imaging method of choice for diagnosis of cholangitis.

Primary sclerosing cholangitis

Primary sclerosing cholangitis (PSC) is a chronic cholestatic liver disease of unknown aetiology. It is characterized by inflammation, destruction, and fibrosis of intrahepatic and extrahepatic bile ducts[15,16]. Ultrasound criteria for the diagnosis of PSC include segmental intrahepatic bile duct dilatation, wall thickening, layering of the CBD, strong reflexes from intrahepatic ducts, and enlarged lymph nodes at the liver hilus[16,17]. Facultative criteria encompass biliary sludge and debris, and rarely CBS stenosis. The diagnostic value of ultrasound is that of a screening method, which provides supplementary information about stage, complications, and follow-up of PSC. ERCP is still the gold standard for diagnosis of PSC, whereas MRCP may become the method of choice in the future. Primary biliary cirrhosis (PBC) is also a chronic inflammatory, cholestatic liver disease. In contrast to PSC, PBC involves the small intrahepatic bile ducts, which cannot be visualized by ultrasound. Therefore, ultrasound may only detect indirect signs of cirrhosis in such patients.

Cholangiocarcinoma

Cholangiocarcinoma is classified into three types: (1) peripheral cholangiocarcinoma, which involves the small intrahepatic bile ducts; (2) hilar cholangiocarcinoma (Klatskin's tumour); and (3) bile duct carcinoma, which involves the extrahepatic bile duct. Peripheral cholangiocarcinoma is usually solitary; it has no specific ultrasound features but may present as a lesion with a halo. Ultrasound is of little value for specific diagnosis of such patients. It is used as a screening method and for follow-up. Diagnosis is verified by ultrasound-guided fine-needle biopsy. Klatskin's tumour typically presents with dilated intrahepatic bile ducts, whereas the tumour lesion itself can rarely be seen. Diagnosis is made by ERCP combined with biopsy and cytology. Endoscopic ultrasound-guided biopsy provides another novel diagnostic procedure[18,19]. Extrahepatic bile duct carcinoma is characterized by focal wall thickening and bile duct dilation. Ultrasound directs management in such patients, but ERCP and biopsy are the diagnostic gold standard. Early diagnosis of cholangiocarcinoma is difficult and has not been achieved in most cases. Recently, a novel miniature ultrasonic imaging system for intraluminal application in the biliary system has become available, named IDUS (intraductal ultrasound). This technique takes advantage of a high-frequency ultrasound miniprobe, which can be introduced into the biliary system through the working channel of conventional duodenoscopes. The transducer frequency varies between 12.5 and 30 MHz. This methodology enables the visualization of the bile duct wall and the adjacent tissue and can be advanced up to segment branches. It is hoped that IDUS will improve the diagnosis of extrahepatic and hilar cholangiocarcinoma[20].

CONCLUSIONS

Ultrasound is the imaging method of choice for directing the management of jaundiced patients and patients with suspected biliary disease. Ultrasound is the gold standard in the diagnosis of gallbladder pathologies, such as gallstones, cholecystitis, gallbladder polyps and porcelain gallbladder. In addition, ultrasound is the primary screening procedure of bile ducts that allows for detection of biliary obstruction, cholangitis and carcinoma. Future developments include intraductal ultrasound with high-resolution miniprobes, three-dimensional ultrasound and endoscopic ultrasound with electronic radial scanners. It is hoped that these innovations will further improve the management of patients with biliary disease.

References

1. Cooperberg PL, Gibney RG. Imaging of the gallbladder, 1987. Radiology. 1987;163:605–13.
2. Lindsell DR. Ultrasound imaging of pancreas and biliary tract. Lancet. 1990;335:390–3.
3. Bennett WF, Bova JG. Review of hepatic imaging and a problem-oriented approach to liver masses. Hepatology. 1990;12:761–75.
4. Wagner S, Gebel M, Bleck JS, Manns MP. Clinical application of three-dimensional sonography in hepatobiliary disease. Bildgebung. 1994;61:104–9.
5. Benson MD, Gandhi MR. Ultrasound of the hepatobiliary–pancreatic system. World J Surg. 2000;24:166–70.
6. Simanowski J. Cholecystolithiasis. In: Gebel M, ed, Ultrasound in Gastroenterology and Hepatology. Berlin Vienna: Blackwell Science, 2000:102–3.
7. Pedersen OM, Nordgard K, Kvinnsland S. Value of sonography in obstructive jaundice. Limitations of bile duct caliber as an index of obstruction. Scand J Gastroenterol. 1987;22:975–81.
8. Partanen KP, Pikkarainen PH, Alhava EM, Janatuinen EK, Pirinen AE. A comparison of ultrasound, computed tomography and endoscopic retrograde cholangiopancreatography in the differential diagnosis of benign and malignant jaundice and cholestasis. Eur J Surg. 1993;159:23–9.
9. Harvey RT, Miller WT Jr. Acute biliary disease: initial CT and follow-up US versus initial US and follow-up CT. Radiology. 1999;213:831–6.
10. Vilgrain V, Palazzo L. Choledocholithiasis: role of US and endoscopic ultrasound. Abdom Imaging. 2001;26:7–14.
11. Collett JA, Allan RB, Chisholm RJ, Wilson IR, Burt MJ, Chapman BA. Gallbladder polyps: prospective study. J Ultrasound Med. 1998;17:207–11.
12. Wibbenmeyer LA, Sharafuddin MJ, Wolverson MK, Heiberg EV, Wade TP, Shields JB. Sonographic diagnosis of unsuspected gallbladder cancer: imaging findings in comparison with benign gallbladder conditions. Am J Roentgenol. 1995;165:1169–74.
13. Mizuguchi M, Kudo S, Fukahori T *et al*. Endoscopic ultrasonography for demonstrating loss of multiple-layer pattern of the thickened gallbladder wall in the preoperative diagnosis of gallbladder cancer. Eur Radiol. 1997;7:1323–7.
14. Wagner S. Infectious cholangitis. In: Gebel M, ed, Ultrasound in Gastroenterology and Hepatology. Berlin Vienna: Blackwell Science, 2000:116–17.
15. Lee YM, Kaplan MM. Primary sclerosing cholangitis. N Engl J Med. 1995;332:924–33.
16. Wagner S, Maschek H, Meier PN, Nashan B, Manns MP. Aktuelle Diagnostik der primär sklerosierenden Cholangitis. Dtsch Med Wochenschr. 1998;123:291–5.

17. Wagner S. Autoimmune cholangitis. In: Gebel M, ed, Ultrasound in Gastroenterology and Hepatology. Berlin Vienna: Blackwell Science, 2000:118–19.
18. Fritscher-Ravens A, Broering DC et al. EUS-guided fine-needle aspiration cytodiagnosis of hilar cholangiocarcinoma: a case series. Gastrointest Endosc. 2000;52:534–40.
19. Bentz JS, Kochman ML, Faigel DO, Ginsberg GG, Smith DB, Gupta PK. Endoscopic ultrasound-guided real-time fine-needle aspiration: clinicopathologic features of 60 patients. Diagn Cytopathol. 1998;18:98–109.
20. Tamada K, Kanai N, Wada S et al. Utility and limitations of intraductal ultrasonography in distinguishing longitudinal cancer extension along the bile duct from inflammatory wall thickening. Abdom Imaging. 2001;26:623–31.

18
Diagnostic approach to unclear liver tumours

J. SCHÖLMERICH

INTRODUCTION

Due to the wide distribution of ultrasound examinations in daily practice the number of focal liver lesions detected has increased significantly in the past two decades[1]. Since this situation increases patients' fears, fast and cost-effective diagnostic approaches to clarify the status of the lesion are necessary[2]. This chapter aims to describe the situations most frequently encountered, and to provide algorithms for the work-up.

SIZE OF THE PROBLEM

There are many different focal liver lesions. Among the benign epithelial lesions adenoma is probably the most common. Among the malignant lesions derived from epithelial tissue metastases and hepatocellular carcinoma are most frequent. Haemangioma is the most important of the benign non-epithelial tumours; metastases can also be derived from non-epithelial origins. Finally tumour-like lesions are frequent, and dysontogenic cysts and focal nodular hyperplasia dominate (Figure 1).

A study describing 75 840 ultrasound examinations revealed 1781 liver lesions. Among the 1382 'solid lesions' the vast majority were metastases of known tumours. A total of 180 lesions remained unclear and were worked up further (Figure 2)[3]. Of the 180 solid lesions about a third were metastases of unknown primary tumours; cysts and haemangiomas were the other major groups (Figure 3). Another study assessed the frequency of benign hepatic lesions detected incidentally using portal venous phase computerized tomography (CT) scans. Of the 1892 patients undergoing tomography during 14 months 100 patients could be included who did not have malignant diseases, liver

UNCLEAR LIVER TUMOURS

Malignant epithelial
Metastases
HCC
Cholangiolar carcinoma
Carcinoid
Others

Malignant nonepithelial
Metastases
Lymphoma
Epitheloid hemangio-
endothelioma
Sarcoma

Benign epithelial
Adenoma
Biliary cystadenoma

Benign nonepithelial
Hemangioma
Lipoma
Angiomyolipoma
Infantile hemangio-
endothelioma

Tumour like lesions
Dysontogenic cysts
Posttraumatic lesions
Echinococcus
Abscesses
FNH
FRH
Focal steatosis
Peliosis
Caroli syndrome

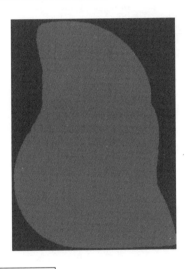

Figure 1 Aetiological classification of focal liver lesions

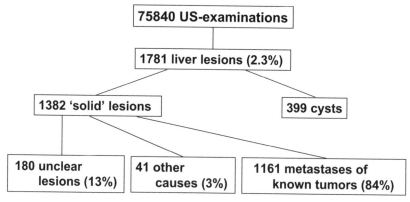

Figure 2 Liver lesions detected in a large ultrasound series[3]

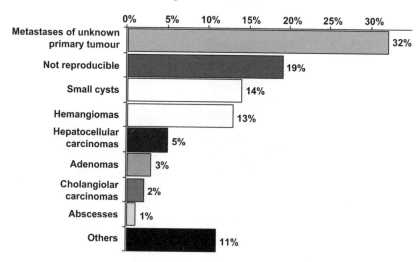

Figure 3 Aetiological classification of 180 solid liver lesions initially found by ultrasound[3]

cirrhosis, or a prior suspicion of a focal lesion. In 33 of these 100 patients 108 lesions were detected. Eighty cysts were found in 14 patients, 18 haemangiomas in 11, and 10 other lesion in nine patients. The average size of the lesions[4] was 9.4 mm with a range of 3–30 mm.

GOALS OF IMAGING WITH UNCLEAR LIVER TUMOURS

There are three different situations which should be distinguished regarding the work-up of an unclear liver lesion. The first comprises patients with non-malignant tumours in whom, during staging procedures or during follow-up, a liver lesion is detected. The second situation relates to the accidental finding of a liver lesion in an otherwise healthy person without known malignancy[1]. A similar problem occurs in patients with liver cirrhosis in whom 'lesions' or nodules are detected.

PATIENTS WITH KNOWN MALIGNANT TUMOURS

Figure 4 describes the goals of imaging in such patients. Depending on the specific problem either high specificity, high sensitivity, or both are required. The imaging modalities available differ with regard to their sensitivity, specificity, detection limit (size of the lesion), and costs. CT and magnetic resonance imaging (MRI) have the highest specificity, CT has probably the best sensitivity (Table 1)[5-10]. There are only a few studies systematically comparing different imaging modalities using a gold standard such as surgery and intraoperative ultrasound, and performing a lesion-by-lesion analysis which is necessary to really compare the capabilities of these techniques. One such study, published in the late 1980s, found CT with arterial and portal contrast (CTAP) to be the best (Table 2)[11]. Meanwhile probably the new spiral CT techniques, allowing visualization during different contrast phases, are probably as good as CTAP, but

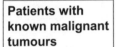

| Patients with known malignant tumours | 1 ⟶ Classification of lesion prior to surgery of the primary (curative versus palliative approach) |

2 ⟶ Classification of lesion with suspected distant recurrence (treatment versus no treatment)

3 ⟶ Exclusion of multiple lesions (surgery versus chemotherapy)

⟹ High specificity (1+2) and high sensitivity (3)

Figure 4 Goals of imaging with unclear liver tumors I

Table 1 Characteristics of imaging modalities for the detection of focal liver lesions

	US	CT	MRI	RN scan
Detection limit (cm)	0.5–2.0	0.8–2.0	0.8–2.0	>2.0
Sensitivity (%)	50–70	57–90	54–80	40–60
Specificity (%)	90	>95	>95	>95
Additional information	+	+	+	−
Cost	Low	Medium	High	Medium

Table 2 Detection of small liver lesions with different imaging modalities[11]

Size	Native CT	Delayed CT	CTAP	MRI
<1 cm	0/18 (0%)	0/9 (0%)	11/18 (61%)	3/18 (17%)
1–2 cm	2/6 (33%)	3/5 (60%)	6/6 (100%)	5/6 (83%)
>2 cm	12/13 (93%)	9/9 (100%)	13/13 (100%)	13/13 (100%)
Total	14/37 (38%)	12/23 (52%)	30/37 (81%)	21/37 (57%)

MEDICAL IMAGING IN GASTROENTEROLOGY AND HEPATOLOGY

Table 3 Doppler ultrasound modalities for differentiation of 133 hepatic lesions[17]

Colour and power doppler	→ (Cutoff)	No specific diagnostic vascular patterns	Accuracy (%)
Peak frequency	(1320 Hz)	HCC vs. MRN	92.6
Resistive index	(0.65)	Malignant vs. benign	83.8
Systolic acceleration time	(105 ms)	HCC vs. metastases	80.9

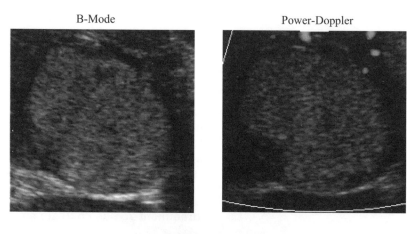

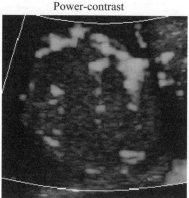

Figure 5 Application of tissue harmonic imaging and contrast-power mode to a liver lesion (initially haemangioma, finally hepatocellular carcinoma)

to our knowledge this has not been studied systematically. For the exclusion of multiple lesions spiral CT is therefore probably the method of choice. It may well be that the novel ultrasound techniques such as harmonic imaging, Doppler modalities, and in particular contrast sonography are equally effective, but this also needs further study[12-15].

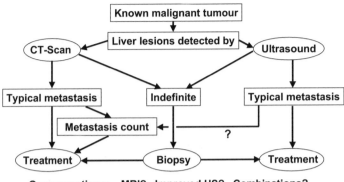

Figure 6 Approach to a liver lesion detected by CT or ultrasound in patients with known malignant tumours

Regarding the classification of a lesion, again very few studies are available. Thus far ultrasound or CT-guided biopsy may still be the best way. A study by Fornari et al.[16] described ultrasound-guided biopsy in 385 patients with lesions of less than 3 cm in diameter; 61% were smaller than 1 cm and 36% between 1 and 2 cm. Histology revealed 135 hepatocellular carcinomas (HCC), 97 metastases, and 11 lymphomas. The specificity was, as expected, 100%, and the sensitivity 86%. More recently Doppler ultrasound modalities were tested for the ability to differentiate hepatic lesions. While colour and power Doppler did not reveal any specific diagnostic vascular patterns, peak frequency, resistive index and systolic acceleration time could be used for differentiation of specific entities (Table 3)[17]. Figure 5 gives an example of a HCC defined by power mode contrast sonography.

Regarding this first situation of a liver lesion detected in a patient with a known malignant tumour, based on the available data the algorithm shown in Figure 6 can be followed. If CT or ultrasound define a typical metastasis, CT will be used for the metastasis count if this is of any importance for treatment decisions – for example surgical removal of metastases. Otherwise treatment can be based upon the initial imaging procedure. In those patients in whom ultrasound or CT detect lesions which are indefinite, a biopsy is the easiest way to achieve diagnosis, and this then can lead to treatment. At this time it is unclear if MRI or the new ultrasound modalities, or any combination, may be superior to this approach.

ACCIDENTALLY FOUND LESIONS WITHOUT KNOWN MALIGNANCY

In this situation the goals are exclusion of malignancy and classification of non-malignant lesions, since both questions are relevant regarding treatment (Figure 7). The most important and frequent lesions have different characteristics in different

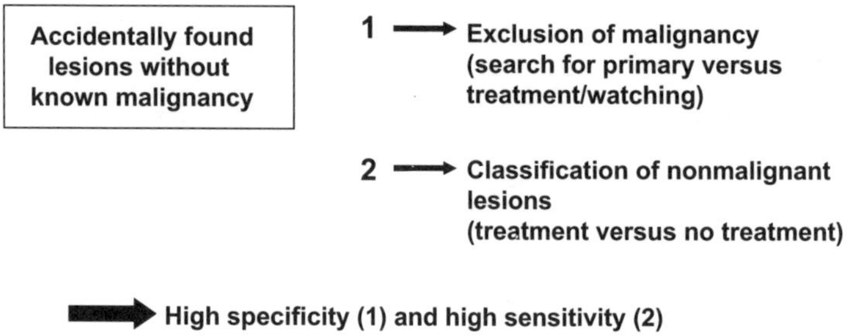

Accidentally found lesions without known malignancy

1 ⟶ Exclusion of malignancy (search for primary versus treatment/watching)

2 ⟶ Classification of nonmalignant lesions (treatment versus no treatment)

⟹ High specificity (1) and high sensitivity (2)

Figure 7 Goals of imaging with unclear liver tumours II

Table 4 Characteristics of liver lesions in imaging modalities

Lesion	Gold standard	US	CD-US	CT	MRI	RN Scan
Haemangioma	US (90%)	Echogenic	?	+ (90%)	+	(+)
Cyst	US	Echofree	—	(+)	—	—
Adenoma	Biopsy	?	—	?	?	Colloid (90%)
FNH	CT/RNS	(+)	+	'Blush'	(+)	HBS:+
Metastasis	Biopsy	(+)	(+)	+	(+)	—
HCC	Biopsy	(+)	?	(+)	?	—

imaging modalities (Table 4)[1,2,8–10]. Regarding the exclusion of malignancy, again modern CT technology may be the best first approach. However, novel ultrasound technologies should not be overlooked. Contrast ultrasound sonography reveals very similar pictures to contrast CT (Figures 8 and 9) but little information from controlled studies is available at present. Biopsy may still be required for exclusion of malignancy in some lesions.

Regarding the classification of non-malignant lesions CT techniques are again the dominant standard, but the application of novel ultrasound technologies may change this situation in the near future. Radionuclide scan still has a limited role in the differentiation of FNH and adenoma when CT or contrast ultrasound sonography are unequivocal. Typical haemangiomas and typical cysts can be defined by ultrasound and need no further imaging. Figure 10 gives an algorithm for the work-up of accidental liver lesions found by ultrasound.

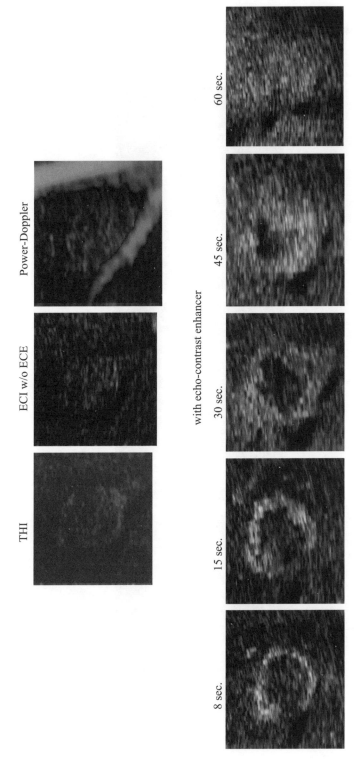

Figure 8 Typical appearance of haemangioma without contrast and with contrast in ultrasound: increasing contrast from the rim to the centre

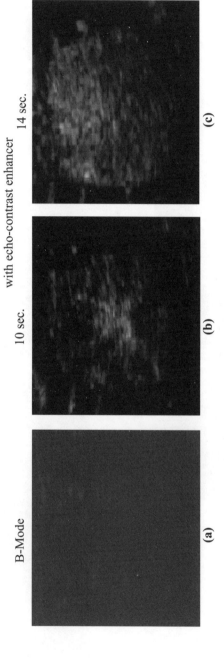

Figure 9 Focal nodular hyperplasia in standard ultrasonography (**a**), tissue harmonic imaging mode (**b**), and contrast burst (**c**)

UNCLEAR LIVER TUMOURS

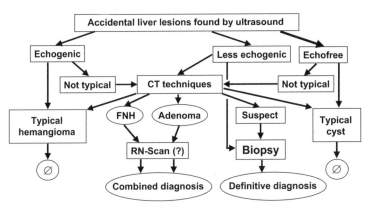

Figure 10 Approach to liver lesions accidentally found by ultrasound

LESIONS OR NODULES IN LIVER CIRRHOSIS

In patients with liver cirrhosis the detection of a nodule or a 'lesion' raises the problem of surgical treatment, liver transplantation or observation (Figure 11). Since it is known that metastases of colorectal carcinoma are rare in cirrhosis and 'non-malignant' regenerating nodules are frequent, but transformation into hepatocellular carcinoma is possible over short time intervals, clarification of this situation is urgent. Depending on the region HCC is more or less frequent, which may be the cause of different results from screening models in different regions of the world[18–21]. Neither initial α-fetoprotein (AFP), ultrasound characteristics nor initial extranodular dysplasia is able to distinguish nodules undergoing transformation into malignant lesions or not from each other, although there are trends regarding echogenicity in ultrasound, frequency of dysplasia and initial 'typical' appearance[22] (Table 5). However, as mentioned above, screening approaches using AFP and ultrasound have widely different sensitivity and specificity, and accordingly have very variable relevance in different studies[18,20] (Table 6; Figure 12). A number of indicators of malignancy have been proposed such as portal thrombus or 'pseudocapsule' in CT, and peak frequency in Doppler sonography. However, their real value is not known at present. Biopsy is also rather difficult, since in many patients multiple nodules are present and it is not clear which one should be biopsied, or how many biopsies should be taken. Interestingly, a recent study describes that a significant number of HCC was detected in small nodules which were seen only by ultrasound, but not by

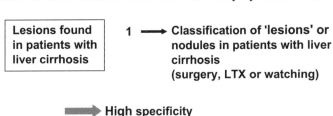

Figure 11 Goals of imaging with unclear liver tumors III

Table 5 Macronodules in liver cirrhosis[22]

26 Months observation	Transformed (n = 8)	Not transformed (n = 24)
Initial AFP (ng/ml)	13 ± 9	12 ± 14
US		
Echogenic (n)	5	6
Less echogenic (n)	3	18
Initial extranodular dysplasia (n)	5	6
Initially 'typical' appearance (n)	3	22

Table 6 Characteristics of different screening techniques for HCC[20]

	Sensitivity (%)	Specificity (%)	PPV (%)
US	78	93	73
AFP > 15 ng/ml	21	93	60

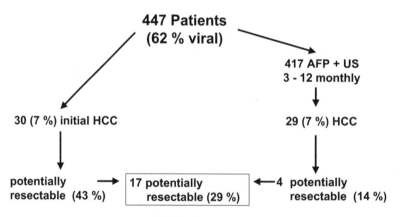

Figure 12 Results of screening for hepatocellular carcinoma in Italian patients with liver cirrhosis[18]

CTAP or DSA[23] (Figure 13). Furthermore most of these nodules, including those with HCC, were not detected by MRI. Thus, at present there is no real algorithm for the approach in patients with lesions in a cirrhotic liver. Neither biopsy, Doppler sonography nor AFP is really helpful. The role of positron emission tomography (PET) is also rather dubious (Figure 14).

SUMMARY

Summarizing the data given above it is obvious that many lesions occur in patients with known malignancy. Bayes' theorem tells us that we should

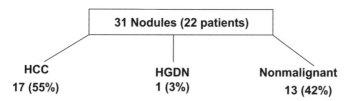

Figure 13 Status of small cirrhotic nodules detected by ultrasound but not by CTAP[23]
MRI = magnetic resonance imaging
HCC = hepatocellular carcinoma
HGDN = high grade dysplastic nodules
DSA = digital subtraction angiography

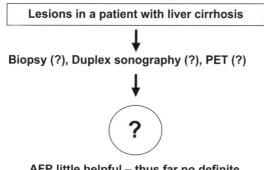

Figure 14 Approach to lesions in patients with liver cirrhosis

therefore use a short approach. If therapeutic implications are lacking no further diagnostics are needed. If decisions have to be made, and findings in either ultrasound or computed tomography are not definitive, biopsies should be taken.

Few lesions occur in patients without risk factors, in particular malignant tumours. Ultrasound characteristics, and in some cases CT, will clarify most of these. Radionuclide scans are not really needed, but may be helpful in some cases where distinction between FNH and adenoma cannot otherwise be made. Biopsy may be needed for adenoma. Most haemangiomas and cysts can be clarified by ultrasound alone.

There is no really convincing approach for lesions detected in cirrhotic livers. For all three situations novel ultrasound technologies may change the algorithm.

Consideration of possible therapeutic consequences seems to be the major intellectual challenge in all described situations, and may be able to avoid most of the multistep diagnostic situations.

References

1. Schölmerich J. Problem: Sonographisch auffällige Leber. In: Schölmerich J, Bischoff SC, Manns MP, eds. Diagnostik in der Gastroenterologie und Hepatologie. Stuttgart: Thieme, 1997:146–50.
2. Feuerbach S. Computertomographie bei Erkrankungen der parenchymatösen Organe des Oberbauchs – Leber, Pankreas, Milz. Internist. 1993;34:229–41.
3. Weiss H. Probleme bei der Diagnostik von Raumforderungen der Leber. In: Gebel M, Majewski A, Brunkhorst R, eds. Sonographie in der Gastroenterologie. Berlin: Springer, 1987:89–90.
4. Völk M, Strotzer M, Lenhart M, Techert J, Seitz J, Feuerbach S. Frequency of benign hepatic lesions incidentally detected with contrast-enhanced thin-section portal venous phase spiral CT. Acta Radiol. 2001;42:172–5.
5. Grebe P, Schild H, Kreitner KF. Differenzierung zwischen benignen und malignen Leberläsionen mit der Nativ-MRT. Fortschr Röntgenstr. 1994;161:412–16.
6. Hamm B, Thoeni RF, Gould RG. Focal liver lesions: characterization with non-enhanced and dynamic contrast material-enhanced MR imaging. Radiology. 1994;190:417–23.
7. Honda H, Onitsuka H, Murakami J. Characteristic findings of hepatocellular carcinoma: an evaluation with comparative study of US, CT, and MRI. Gastrointest Radiol. 1992;17:245–9.
8. Soyer P, Bluemke DA, Hruban RH, Sitzmann JV, Fishmann EK. Primary malignant neoplasms of the liver: detection with helical CT during arterial portography. Radiology. 1994;192:389–92.
9. Soyer P, Bluemke DA, Fishmann EK. CT during arterial portography for the preoperative evaluation of hepatic tumors: How, when and why? Am J Radiol. 1994;164:1325–31.
10. Soyer P, Laissy JP, Sibert A. Focal hepatic masses. Comparison of detection during arterial portography with MR imaging and CT. Radiology. 1994;190:737–40.
11. Heiken J, Weymann PJ, Lee JKT. Detection of focal hepatic masses: prospective evaluation with CT, delayed CT, CT during arterial portography, and MR imaging. Radiology. 1989;171:47–51.
12. Chen RC, Wand CS, Chen PH. Carbon dioxide-enhanced ultrasonography of liver tumors. Ultrasound Med. 1994;13:81–6.
13. Fujimoto M, Moriysu F, Nishikawa K. Color doppler sonography of hepatic tumors with a galactose-based contrast agent: correlation with angiographic findings. Am J Radiol. 1994;163:1099–104.
14. Kubo S, Kinoshita H, Hirohashi K. Preoperative localization of hepatomas by sonography with microbubbles of carbon dioxide. Am J Radiol. 1994;163:1405–6.
15. Reinhold C, Hammers L, Taylor CR. Characterization of local lesions with duplex sonography: findings in 198 patients. Am J Radiol. 1995;164:1131–5.
16. Fornari F, Filice C, Rapaccini GL. Small (≤ 3 cm) hepatic lesions. Results of sonographically fine-needle biopsy in 385 patients. Dig Dis Sci. 1994;39:2267–75.
17. Gaiani S, Casali A, Serr C et al. Assessment of vascular patterns of small liver mass lesions: value and limitation of the different Doppler ultrasound modalities. Am J Gastroenterol. 2000;95:3537–46.
18. Colombo M, de Franchis R, Del Ninno E et al. Hepatocellular carcinoma in Italian patients with cirrhosis. N Engl J Med. 1991;325:675–80.
19. Miller WJ, Baron RL, Dodd GD. Malignancies in patients with cirrhosis: CT sensitivity and specificity in 200 consecutive transplant patients. Radiology. 1994;193:643–50.
20. Pateron D, Ganne N, Trincet JS. Prospective study of screening for hepatocellular carcinoma in Caucasian patients with cirrhosis. J Hepatol. 1994;20:65–71.
21. Rizzi PM, Kane PA, Ryder SD. Accuracy of radiology in detection of hepatocellular carcinoma before liver transplantation. Gastroenterology. 1994;107:1425–29.
22. Borzio M, Borzio F, Croce A et al. Ultrasonography-detected macroregenerative nodules in cirrhosis: a prospective study. Gastroenterology. 1997;112:1617–23.
23. Tanaka Y, Sasaki Y, Katayama K et al. Probability of hepatocellular carcinoma of small hepatocellular nodules undetectable by computed tomography during arterial portography. Hepatology. 2000;31:890–8.

Section VII
Imaging – new technologies

19
Fluorescence endoscopy in gastroenterology

H. MESSMANN and E. ENDLICHER

BACKGROUND

The detection of early-stage cancer is one of the major goals in medicine, in particular in gastrointestinal endoscopy. Barrett's oesophagus, ulcerative colitis and other premalignant conditions are associated with an increased cancer risk and regular surveillance endoscopies are recommended[1,2].

Adenocarcinoma in Barrett's oesophagus or ulcerative colitis arises from dysplasia, which is usually not visible during routine endoscopy[3]. Because of the multistep neoplastic progression in developing cancer, and the excellent therapeutic modalities in superficial growth stages without metastasis, an early diagnosis of precancerous lesions would be of essential benefit for individuals with long-standing and extensive ulcerative colitis, Barrett's oesophagus or other premalignant conditions.

The most significant predictor of the risk of malignancy in patients with inflammatory bowel disease is the presence of dysplasia in colonic biopsies. Prevalence of dysplasia in ulcerative colitis ranges from 4%[4] to 13%[5] for high-grade dysplasia and 26% for low-grade dysplasia[6].

The precancerous lesions and cancers associated with ulcerative colitis usually present as flat or infiltrative lesions with no or only non-specific macroscopic characteristics. Furthermore a positive histological finding in a normal-appearing mucosa often is a not reproducible diagnosis, since this area cannot be exactly localized in a control examination[7].

Therefore extensive random sampling of the entire Barrett's segment or colon should be performed with biopsies in the four quadrants every 1–2 cm or 10 cm, respectively, and of any macroscopic abnormalities. Nevertheless, these random biopsies are associated with an inevitable sampling error[2]. To detect dysplasia in ulcerative colitis with a probability of 90% at least 33 random biopsies are necessary[8].

New technical methods have been developed to resolve this problem. Fluorescence endoscopy, chromoendoscopy, light-scattering spectroscopy and optical coherence tomography may play important roles. Fluorescence endoscopy includes either laser-induced fluorescence spectroscopy (LIFS) or laser/light-induced fluorescence endoscopy (LIFE). Both techniques use exogenous or endogenous fluorophores to detect the tissue fluorescence.

PRINCIPLE OF FLUORESCENCE DIAGNOSIS

The principle of fluorescence diagnosis is based on the interaction of light and tissue. Irradiation of tissue with light of a specific wavelength leads to excitation of endogenous or exogenous fluorophores causing electrons to be raised to a higher energy level. Subsequent relaxation induces emission of a typical fluorescence light.

ENDOGENOUS TISSUE AUTOFLUORESCENCE

Among these endogenous fluorophores coenzymes play an important role: NADH, flavin, collagen, elastin and porphyrin. A shift to the oxidized forms such as for NAD, NADP, FAD and FMN results in a lack of fluorescence, while collagen, elastin and porphyrins have a typical excitation and emission spectrum (Table 1). Different excitation wavelengths will result in activation of different fluorophores. A number of processes such as inflammation, ischaemia, but also dysplasia influence the metabolic and oxidative status of the cells, and therefore the autofluorescence of the tissue. Furthermore, autofluorescence is influenced by the thickness of the mucosa. The penetration depth of the excitation light at 400 nm is about 500 μm. The average thickness of the mucosa is 460 μm; therefore the collagen and elastin of the mucosa will be excited. A thickening of the mucosa will result in a decreased autofluorescence of elastin and collagen[9].

EXOGENOUS FLUOROPHORES

Among exogenous fluorophores, 5-aminolaevulinic acid (5-ALA) is the most interesting substance for fluorescence diagnosis[10]. It is not a sensitizer itself, but

Table 1 Excitation and emission wavelengths of various fluorophores in tissue. The data represent maximum values at optimum excitation/emission condition

Fluorophores	Excitation (nm)	Emission (nm)
NADH	350	500
Flavin	455	495
Collagen	250	330
Elastin	285	350
Porphyrin	405	610

is converted intracellularly into the photoactive compound protoporphyrin IX (PPIX) (Figure 1). The cellular uptake of 5-ALA is still not clear, but 5-ALA seems to be taken up by an active transport mechanism[11].

PPIX is characterized by a typical absorption band in the ultraviolet region with a characteristic emission in red light. It is associated with a significantly higher tumour selectivity compared with other haematoporphyrins[12]. A reduced ferrochelatase activity is one hypothesis for selective accumulation in malignant tissues. Furthermore the enhanced synthesis catalysed by an increased activity of porphobilinogen deaminase in tumour cells is another possibility for selective accumulation of PPIX[13,14].

In principle almost all cells of the human body, with the exception of mature red blood cells, are able to produce haem and the various porphyrins.

In a number of animal studies it could be demonstrated that PPIX accumulates preferentially in the mucosal epithelium of the aerodigestive tract, urothelium, epidermis and endometrium, but also in the epithelium of the gastrointestinal tract[15-17]. Since there is a high tissue specificity of exogenous 5-ALA-derived porphyrins produced mostly in the mucosal epithelium, but with little specificity in the underlying submucosa and muscle layers in most internal hollow organs. Therefore premalignant and malignant counterparts of the mucosal epithelium in these organs are expected to be promising for PDT with 5-ALA or fluorescence detection.

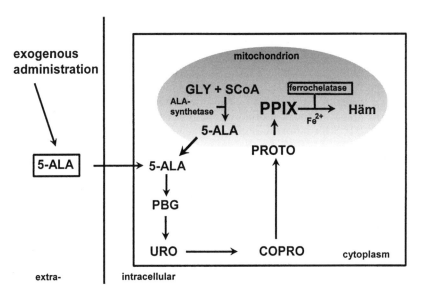

Figure 1 Porphyrin biosynthesis after exogenous application of 5-ALA. There are several possibilities for selectivity of protoporphyrin IX in tumour cells: (1) enhanced cellular uptake of 5-ALA into the cell, (2) enhanced activity of the porphyrin synthesis, (3) reduced activity of the enzyme ferrochelatase. (GLY = glycine; SCoA = succinyl-CoA; 5-ALA = 5-aminolaevulinic acid; PBG = porphobilinogen; URO = uroporphyrinogen; COPRO = coproporphyrinogen; PROTO = protoporphyrinogen; PPIX = protoporphyrin IX)

The detection of tumours within normal tissue depends on the ratio of PPIX in malignant and normal tissue. The ratio itself is a function of the used 5-ALA dose and the time delay between sensitization and examination, and is ideally about 1:6. Furthermore, skin sensitivity is reduced to 24–48 hours, which might be even lower or not present after local sensitization[18–20].

ENDOSCOPIC FLUORESCENCE DETECTION

Spectroscopy

Laser-induced fluorescence spectroscopy (LIFS) is a very interesting method to differentiate tissue without taking biopsies and using histological features, and could play a beneficial role in the detection of precancerous lesions in Barrett's oesophagus. With this technique laser light is directed via a fibre which is inserted through the biopsy channel of an endoscope to the tissue examined. The fluorescence emitted from the tissue is collected either by the same fibre or by separate fibres. A fluorescence spectrometer with a sensitive detector records the fluorescence signal, dependent on the wavelength of the exciting light, but also on biological and physicochemical properties of the examined tissue. In a number of trials LIFS was able to differentiate malignant from benign lesions such as colon cancer from adenomatous polyps and hyperplastic polyps (Table 2).

Panjehpour and co-workers used a differential normalized fluorescence index technique to differentiate high-grade dysplasia (HGD) from either low-grade or non-dysplastic mucosa. With this technique 36 patients were examined and 96% of non-dysplastic Barrett's oesophagus samples were correctly classified as benign, all low-grade dysplasia (LGD) as benign and 90% of the HGD as premalignant[23].

Stael von Holstein et al. used the combination of exogenous and endogenous fluorophores to discriminate LGD, HGD and adenocarcinoma from normal oesophageal and gastric mucosa by LIFS[24]. Patients were sensitized with low doses of Photofrin© (0.35 mg/kg i.v.) and fluorescence intensity ratios at 630 nm (Photofrin©) and 500 nm (autofluorescence) were calculated. The mean values were 0.1 ± 0.058 for normal oesophageal mucosa, 0.16 ± 0.073 for normal gastric mucosa, 0.205 ± 0.17 for Barrett's epithelium with moderate dysplasia, 0.79 ± 0.54 for severe dysplasia, and 0.78 ± 0.56 for adenocarcinoma. Thus differentiation of early cancers as well as HGD from LGD or normal mucosa in Barrett's oesophagus was possible with this technique. One disadvantage of LIFS using autofluorescence is the enormous costs for the highly sophisticated systems. Furthermore, up to now differentiation of different tissues is possible only by optical spectroscopy using point measurements. With this technique suspicious lesions must first be detected by visual inspection. To detect non-visible dysplasia in Barrett's oesophagus point measurements are necessary which are comparable to random biopsies and are still associated with unavoidable 'sampling error'.

Fluorescence endoscopy

Fluorescence endoscopy after sensitization with 5-ALA is another promising method for detection of precancerous lesions in the gastrointestinal tract[10].

Table 2 LIFS in gastrointestinal tumours

Main author/ref.	Excitation wavelength (nm)	Light source	Detection spectrum (nm)	Fluorescence	Tissue	Sensitivity/specificity/ positive predictive value
Vo-Dinh 1995[21]	410	N2-Laser	430–720	Autofluorescence	Oesophageal cancer (in vivo)	100%/98%/n.d.
Panjehpour 1995[22]	410	N2-Laser	430–716	Autofluorescence	Oesophageal cancer (in vivo)	100%/98%/–
Panjehpour 1996[23]	410	N2-Laser	430–716	Autofluorescence	Barrett's oesophagus–dysplasia (in vivo)	90%/96%/–
Stael von Holstein 1996[24]	405	N2-Laser	450–750	Quotient: Porphyrin-/Autofluorescence	Barrett's oesophagus–carcinoma/dysplasia (in vivo + in vitro)	78%/92%/82% (ratio > 0.375 54%/100%/100% ratio > 0.55
Kapadia 1990[25]	325	HeCa-Laser	325–600	Autofluorescence	Colon polyps (in vitro)	100%/99%/98%
Cothren 1990[26]	370	N2-Laser	460–680	Autofluorescence	Colon polyps (in vivo)	100%/97%/94%
Schomacker 1992[27]	337	N2-Laser	300–800	Autofluorescence	Colon polyps and cancer (in vivo)	80%/92%/82%
Eker 1999[28]	337 405 435	N2-Laser (337 nm) Dye laser (405/435 nm)	400–700	Autofluorescence, Porphyrin IX fluorescence	Colon polyps (in vivo)	100%/96%/93%/100% (exogenous + endogenous)

In contrast to spectroscopy, which differentiates malignant and benign lesions, fluorescence endoscopy allows optical guided biopsies, due to selective fluorescence of malignant tissue.

In a DSS colitis model in rats we were able for the first time to visualize dysplasia in colitis after sensitization with 5-ALA. Sensitivity and specificity to detect dysplasia varied with the drug dose used (Table 3)[29].

In patients with Barrett's oesophagus and ulcerative colitis it could be demonstrated that detection of low and/or high grade dysplasia not visible during routine endoscopy were detectable (ich habe was rausgestrichen, bitte diesen Satz noch mal lesen).

In 47 patients with Barrett's oesophagus, 10 of them with known dysplasia, 58 fluorescence endoscopies were performed after sensitization with different concentrations of 5-ALA given orally (5, 10, 20, 30 mg/kg) or locally (500–1000 mg) by spraying the mucosa via a catheter. Fluorescence endoscopy was performed 4–6 h after systemic and 1–2 h after local sensitization using a special light source delivering white or blue light[20]. A total of 243 biopsies of red fluorescent ($n = 113$) and non-fluorescent areas ($n = 30$) were taken. In three patients, two early cancers and dysplasia, not visible during routine endoscopy, were detected by fluorescence endoscopy. Thirty-three biopsies revealed either LGD or HGD. Sensitivity to detect dysplastic lesions ranged from 60% after local sensitization with 500 mg to 80%, 100% and 100% after systemic application of 10, 20 and 30 mg/kg, respectively. However, specificity was best for local sensitization with 70% while systemic administration revealed values between 27% and 56% (Table 4). Using 5 mg/kg no red fluorescence in dysplastic lesions was found. No severe side-effects were noted.

Table 3 Sensitivity and specificity for fluorescence detection of dysplasia in a rat colitis model[29]

5-ALA dose (mg/kg i.v.)	Sensitivity (%)	Specificity (%)
50	42	56
75	92	35
100	100	22

Table 4 Sensitivity, specificity, positive and negative predictive value per biopsies to detect dysplastic lesions in Barrett's oesophagus after different sensitization forms using 5-aminolevulinic acid (5-ALA)[20]

5-ALA application mode	Examinations (biopsies) (n)	Sensitivity (%)	Specificity (%)	Positive predictive value (%)	Negative predictive value (%)
500 mg locally	22 (96)	60	69	18	94
5 mg/kg orally	4 (20)	—	70	0	100
10 mg/kg orally	13 (56)	80	56	40	88
20 mg/kg orally	13 (44)	100	51	13	100
30 mg/kg orally	6 (27)	100	27	23	100

Table 5 Sensitivity and specificity of fluorescence endoscopy in the detection of dysplasia in ulcerative colitis[19]

ALA dose	Examinations (n)	Sensitivity (%)	Specificity (%)
3000 mg locally (enema)	32	87	51
3000 mg locally (spray catheter)	10	100	62
20 mg/kg orally	12	43	73

Gossner et al. examined 35 patients with upper gastrointestinal dysplasia and early cancer. Three hours after sensitization with 10 mg/kg 5-ALA patients were examined with the equipment from Storz, as mentioned above. Neoplasia was detected with a sensitivity and specificity of 85% and 70%, respectively[30]. Another important indication for fluorescence endoscopy comprises patients with long-standing ulcerative colitis. Our experience with 54 examinations in 37 patients showed that local administration of 5-ALA is superior to a systemic sensitization with 20 mg/kg, which is obviously too low to achieve an adequate sensitivity. This finding fits with the data from Regula et al., who demonstrated that, in the lower gastrointestinal tract, a higher 5-ALA dose is necessary to obtain reasonable fluorescence intensity[18].

For details of fluorescence endoscopy in patients with ulcerative colitis see Table 5[19].

Haringsma et al. demonstrated excellent results with laser-induced autofluorescence endoscopy (LIFE; Xillix) for detecting precancerous lesions in patients with Barrett's oesophagus. Eighty patients with oesophagus Barrett's were examined, and sensitivity and specificity for detecting HGD and early cancers were 87%[31]. LGD was correctly identified in only 4/22 cases.

CONCLUSION

LIFS and LIFE are both promising techniques to differentiate or detect precancerous lesions such as dysplasia and gastrointestinal malignancies in the gastrointestinal tract. Autofluorescence offers the advantage of no side-effects caused by sensitizers; however, the sensitivity to detect LGD is still low, and the costs for the equipment are high. LIFS allows differentiation of malignant and benign lesions either with endogenous or exogenous induced fluorescence. Exogenous induced fluorescence by application of 5-ALA may be associated with minor side-effects such as limited skin photosensitivity, but sensitivity to detect even LGD, which is important in patients with ulcerative colitis, is higher, and the equipment is cheaper, and is also commercially available for patients in urology.

To optimize fluorescence-guided biopsies by LIFE improvement of the equipment (videoendoscopes), combination of exogenous and endogenous fluorescence and perhaps new sensitizers such as 5-ALA esters are necessary.

Nevertheless, LIFE is still experimental, and randomized trials comparing the gold standard of biopsy sampling in patients with ulcerative colitis or Barrett's oesophagus are necessary.

References

1. Bond JH. Colorectal surveillance for neoplasia: an overview. Gastrointest Endosc. 1999;49: 35–40.
2. Sampliner RE. Practice guidelines on the diagnosis, surveillance, and therapy of Barrett's esophagus. The Practice Parameters Committee of the American College of Gastroenterology. Am J Gastroenterol. 1998;93:1028–32.
3. McArdle JE, Lewin KJ, Randall G et al. Distribution of dysplasia and early invasive carcinoma in Barrett's esophagus. Hum Pathol. 1992;23:479–82.
4. Herbay AV, Herfarth C, Otto H. Cancer and dysplasia in ulcerative colitis: a histologic study of 301 surgical specimen. Z Gastroenterol. 1994:32;382–8.
5. Connell WR, Lennard-Jones JE, Williams CB et al. Factors affecting the outcome of endoscopic surveillance for cancer in ulcerative colitis. Gastroenterology. 1994;107:934–44.
6. Lindberg B, Persson B, Veress B et al. Twenty years' colonoscopic surveillance of patients with ulcerative colitis. Scand J Gastroenterol. 1996;31:1195–204.
7. Herbay AV. Karzinome bei chronisch entzündlichen Darmerkrankungen. Internist. 1998;39: 1024–9.
8. Rubin C, Haggitt R, Burmer G. DNA aneuploidy in colonic biopsies predicts future development of dysplasia in ulcerative colitis. Gastroenterology. 1992;103:1611–20.
9. Messmann H. [Fluorescence endoscopy in gastroenterology] [article in German]. Z Gastroenterol. 2000;38:21–30.
10. Messmann H. 5-Aminolevulinic acid-induced protoporphyrin IX for the detection of gastrointestinal dysplasia. Gastrointest Endosc Clin N Am. 2000;10:497–512.
11. Bermudez Moretti M, Correa Garcia S, Stella C et al. Delta-aminolevulinic acid transport in *Saccharomyces cerevisiae*. Int J Biochem. 1993;25:1917–20.
12. El-Sharabasy MM, el-Waseef AM, Hafez MM et al. Porphyrin metabolism in some malignant diseases. Br J Cancer. 1992:65:409–12.
13. Hinnen P, de Rooij FW, van Velthuysen ML et al. Biochemical basis of 5-aminolaevulinic acid-induced protoporphyrin IX accumulation: a study in patients with (pre)malignant lesions of the oesophagus. Br J Cancer. 1998:78:679–82.
14. Kennedy JC, Pottier RH, Pross DC. Photodynamic therapy with endogenous protoporphyrin IX: basic principles and present clinical experience. J Photochem Photobiol. 1990;6:143–8.
15. Loh CS, Vernon DI, MacRobert A et al. Endogenous porphyrin distribution induced by 5-aminolaevulinic acid in the tissue layers of the gastrointestinal tract. J Photochem Photobiol B. 1993;20:47–54.
16. Peng Q, Berg K, Moan J et al. 5-Aminolevulinic acid-based photodynamic therapy: principles and experimental research. Cancer. 1997;79:2282–308.
17. Ravi B, Regula J, Buonacorsi GA et al. Sensitization and photodynamic therapy of normal pancreas, duodenum and bile ducts in the hamster using 5-aminolevulinic acid. Lasers Med Sci. 1996;11:11–17.
18. Regula J, MacRobert AJ, Gorchein A. Photosensitisation and photodynamic therapy of oesophageal, duodenal, and colorectal tumours using 5 aminolaevulinic acid induced protoporphyrin IX – pilot study. Gut. 1995;36:67–75.
19. Endlicher E, Knüchel R, Schölmerich J et al. Photodynamic diagnosis of dysplasia in longstanding ulcerative colitis after sensitization with 5-aminolevulinic acid. Gastrointest Endosc. 1999;49:AB117.
20. Endlicher E, Knuechel R, Hauser T, Szeimies RM, Schölmerich J, Messmann H. Endoscopic fluorescence detection of low and high grade dysplasia in Barrett's oesophagus using systemic or local 5-aminolaevulinic acid sensitisation. Gut. 2001;48:314–19.
21. Vo-Dinh T, Panjehpour M, Overholt BF, Farris C, Buckley FP 3rd, Sneed R. *In vivo* cancer diagnosis of the esophagus using differential normalized fluorescence (DNF) indices. Laser Surg Med. 1995;16:41–7.
22. Panjehpour M, Overholt BF, Schmidhammer JL, Farris C, Buckley PF, Vo-Dinh T. Spectroscopic diagnosis of esophageal cancer: new classification model, improved measurement system. Gastrointest Endosc. 1995;41:577–81.
23. Panjehpour M, Overholt BF, Vo-Dinh T, Haggitt RC, Edwards DH, Buckley FP 3rd. Endoscopic fluorescence detection of high-grade dysplasia in Barrett's esophagus. Gastroenterology. 1996;111:93–101.

24. Stael von Holstein CS, Nilsson AM, Andersson-Engels S, Willen R, Walther B, Svanberg K. Detection of adenocarcinoma in Barrett's oesophagus by means of laser induced fluorescence. Gut. 1996;39:711–16.
25. Kapadia CR, Cutruzzola FW, O'Brien KM, Stetz ML, Enriquez R, Deckelbaum LI. Laser-induced fluorescence spectroscopy of human colonic mucosa. Gastroenterology. 1990;99:150–7.
26. Cothren RM, Richards-Kortum R, Sivak MV Jr et al. Gastrointestinal tissue diagnosis by laser-induced fluorescence spectroscopy at endoscopy. Gastrointest Endosc. 1990;36:105–11.
27. Schomacker KT, Frisoli JK, Compton CC et al. Ultraviolet laser-induced fluorescence of colonic polyps. Gastroenterology. 1992;102:1155–60.
28. Eker C, Montan S, Jaramillo E et al. Clinical spectral characterisation of colonic mucosal lesions using autofluorescence and delta aminolevulinic acid sensitisation. Gut. 1999;44:511–18.
29. Messmann H, Kullmann F, Wild T et al. Detection of dysplastic lesions by fluorescence in a model of colitis in rats after previous photosensitization with 5-aminolaevulinic acid. Endoscopy. 1998;30:333–8.
30. Gossner L, Stepp H, Sroka R et al. Photodynamic diagnosis (PDD) of high-grade dysplasia and early cancer in Barrett's esophagus using 5-aminolevulinic acid (ALA). Gastroenterology. 1998;114:A136.
31. Haringsma J. Tytgat GNJ. Light-induced fluorescence endoscopy (LIFE) for the *in vivo* detection of colorectal dysplasia. Gastroenterology. 1998;114:A606.

20
Chromoendoscopy
M. I. F. CANTO

INTRODUCTION

Chromoendoscopy or tissue staining is an 'old' endoscopic technique that has been used for decades. It involves the topical application of stains or pigments to improve localization, characterization, or diagnosis[1]. Tissue staining is a general term that refers to the application of stains or pigments by spraying through a catheter. Vital staining is a type of tissue staining that employs vital stains (Table 1). Other types of tissue staining techniques include contrast staining (using indigo carmine) or reactive staining (using Congo red or phenol red). In contrast to tissue staining, endoscopic tattooing refers to injection of dye (such as India ink) through a needle to mark a site for future identification. This discussion will focus only on chromoendoscopy.

Tissue staining is a useful adjunct to endoscopy; the contrast between normal-stained and abnormal-stained epithelium enables the endoscopist to formulate a diagnosis and/or direct biopsies based on a specific reaction or enhancement of surface morphology. Compared to other endoscopic diagnostic modalities, such as optical coherence spectroscopy, light-induced spectroscopy, and fluorescence endoscopy, chromoendoscopy is simple, quick, widely available, inexpensive, and free of adverse effects.

STAIN EQUIPMENT AND GENERAL TECHNIQUE FOR CHROMOENDOSCOPY

Vital staining usually takes only a few minutes to perform and tissue reactions or absorption usually occurs in seconds to minutes. Vital staining requires minimal equipment and reagents are generally available. A special spray catheter (such as Olympus PW-5L, Olympus America, Inc., Melville, New York) is essential for delivery of stain in a fine mist to the mucosa. The reusable catheters can last several years even with routine use in a busy endoscopy unit. A new biopsy channel cap is useful for preventing stain from leaking out. If staining is being performed for cancer surveillance in a patient with biopsy-proven Barrett's oesophagus, a large-channel/therapeutic upper endoscope is required to accommodate the 'jumbo' biopsy forceps. The technique for staining is simple and easy to learn. When spraying in the oesophagus or colon the endoscopist needs to direct the endoscope and catheter tip towards the oesophageal mucosa and use a combination of rotational clockwise–counterclockwise movements with simultaneous withdrawal of the endoscope tip. This will maximize the amount of reagent applied to the epithelium. The interpretation of staining patterns may need to be learned, and requires an understanding of what type of tissue is stained and what is not stained. Increased resolution of mucosal staining pattern can be provided by high-resolution endoscopes or magnification endoscopes (which can magnify by a factor of 35–115×).

SPECIFIC STAINS USED FOR CHROMOENDOSCOPY

Lugol's solution

Lugol's solution is a readily available reagent that contains potassium iodine and iodine, which has an affinity for glycogen in non-keratinized squamous epithelium. Lugol's staining involves dilution of stock solution to 1–2% followed by spraying of 20–50 ml through a spray catheter. Normal squamous epithelium will stain black, dark brown, or green–brown after a few minutes. Abnormal staining pattern (absence of dye uptake) is associated with conditions that result in depletion of glycogen in squamous cells, such as inflammatory change (reflux oesophagitis), dysplasia, or early malignancy.

Lugol's staining is helpful in detecting high-grade dysplasia and early squamous cell cancers of the oesophagus. Unsuspected early oesophageal cancers can be diagnosed in high-risk patients who undergo screening[1]. The diagnostic yield for early cancer in endoscopic screening programmes that have utilized this technique is significant – 5.1–8.2%[1–3]. Squamous cell carcinoma will fail to show the characteristic colour change of adjacent normal mucosa and will be unstained.

Non-squamous mucosa (such as columnar mucosa such as Barrett's oesophagus) should also not pick up Lugol's stain. Lugol's staining has also been used to improve the detection of Barrett's oesophagus[3]. By increasing the demarcation between squamous mucosa (which will stain dark brown) from unstained, pink metaplastic columnar epithelium, Lugol's staining can increase the sensitivity, specificity, and accuracy of endoscopic diagnosis of Barrett's oesophagus to 89%, 93%, and 91%, respectively[4]. Lugol's staining may also be useful in differentiating regenerating squamous epithelium from small areas of residual Barrett's mucosa in patients who have undergone mucosal ablation (e.g. after photodynamic therapy or multipolar electrocoagulation).

The technique involves spraying of 1.5–3% Lugol's solution (or potassium iodide plus iodine) through a special spray or washing catheter that creates a fine mist. An average of 20 ml is used. After several seconds there will be dark brown to black staining of normal squamous mucosa. The areas to target for biopsy are unstained mucosa, particularly confluent, greater than 5 mm, raised or depressed

Table 1 Tissue stains used in chromoendoscopy

Stain type	What is stained	Mechanism of staining	Positive staining	Clinical uses in gastrointestine
Vital stains				
Lugol's solution (iodine + potassium iodide)	Normal glycogen containing squamous cells	Binds iodine in non-keratinized cells	Dark brown	(1) Squamous cell oesophageal cancer (non-staining). (2) Columnar epithelium in the oesophagus, including residual Barrett's oesophagus following mucosal ablation (non-staining). (3) Reflux oesophagitis (non-staining).
Methylene blue (methylthionine chloride)	Small or large intestinal cells or intestinal metaplasia	Active absorption into cells	Blue	(1) Specialized epithelium (intestinal metaplasia) in Barrett's oesophagus*. (2) Intestinal metaplasia in the stomach. (3) Early gastric cancer†. (4) Gastric metaplasia in the duodenum (non-staining). (5) Coeliac and tropical sprue.
Toluidine blue (tolonium chloride or dimethylamino-toluphenazothioni-chloride	Nuclei of columnar (gastric and intestinal-type) cells	Diffuses into cell	Blue	(1) Squamous cell carcinoma of the oesophagus. (2) Gastric or intestinal metaplasia in Barrett's oesophagus.
Reactive stains				
Congo red (biphenylene-naphthadene sulphonic acid)	Acid-containing gastric cells	Acid pH <3.0 results in colour change	Turns red to dark blue or black	(1) Acid-secreting gastric mucosa (including ectopic locations). (2) Gastric cancer (non-staining); may be combined with methylene blue to outline intestinal metaplasia.

Agent	Stains	Mechanism/Appearance	Uses
Phenol red (phenolsulphon-phthalein)	*H. pylori*-infected gastric cells	Alkaline pH (from hydrolysis of urea to NH_3 and CO_2 by urease) results in colour change. Turns yellow to red	Diagnose *Helicobacter pylori* infection (positive colour change) and map its distribution in the stomach.
Contrast stain			
Indigo carmine‡	Cells are not stained	Pools in crevices and valleys between mucosal projections. Blue (indigo)	(1) Colon, gastric, duodenal, oesophageal lesions. (2) Barrett's oesophagus.
Agents for tattooing			
Purified, sterile carbon (Spot)	Injection site	Mark location of a lesion (permanently). Black	Endoscopic tattoo anywhere in the gastrointestinal tract.
India ink	Injection site	Mark location of a lesion (permanently). Black	(1) Location of colon polyps or cancers for subsequent endoscopic or intraoperative identification. (2) Location of the original squamocolumnar junction prior to mucosal ablation of Barrett's oesophagus.

* Methylene blue does not stain non-specialized or gastric metaplasia; specialized columnar epithelium stains blue but highly dysplastic and malignant specialized columnar epithelia in Barrett's oesophagus generally take up little to no dye; low-grade dysplasia in Barrett's oesophagus may or may not take up stain.
† With or without Congo red.
‡ Also used in combination with high-resolution or high-magnification endoscopy; may be used with or without cresyl violet (for early colorectal cancers).

areas. Remember that iodine allergy is a contraindication to Lugol's staining and laryngeal oedema can occur.

Toluidine blue

Toluidine blue (also called tolonium chloride) is a basic dye that stains cellular nuclei. It has been used to identify malignant tissues, which have an increased DNA synthesis and a high nuclear to cytoplasmic ratio. It will stain abnormal tissues blue. It has been used to help screen for early squamous oesophageal cancers in alcohol and tobacco abusers[5] and patients with head and neck cancers[6]. It can also selectively stain gastric cancers and can help discriminate between benign and malignant ulcers[10]. It can stain oesophageal columnar epithelium, such as Barrett's oesophagus, with a sensitivity of 98% and specificity of 80%[7]. Toluidine blue can stain columnar-type mucosa in Barrett's oesophagus but it cannot discriminate between gastric and intestinal metaplasia. Toluidine blue staining is accomplished by spraying 1% acetic acid before and after 1% aqueous solution of toluidine blue.

Methylene blue

Methylene blue is a vital stain taken up by actively absorbing tissues such as small intestinal and colonic epithelium. It does not stain non-absorptive epithelia such as squamous or gastric mucosa. It has recently been used to highlight subtle mucosal changes in the small intestine (e.g. coeliac disease) and colon (flat adenomas and carcinomas). It has been used to positively stain metaplastic absorptive epithelium, such as intestinal-type metaplasia in the stomach[8]. It will not stain non-absorptive epithelium, such as ectopic gastric metaplasia in a background of positive-staining duodenal mucosa. The technique of methylene blue staining was originally described by Japanese investigators for improving the diagnosis of early gastric cancer, either alone or in combination with Congo red dye[9].

Methylene blue staining has also been used in the oesophagus to aid in the detection of Barrett's oesophagus. Barrett's oesophagus is the metaplastic replacement of squamous epithelium in the oesophagus by columnar epithelium, which resembles cells in the gastric fundus, gastric cardia, or intestine. It is the intestinal-type metaplasia or specialized columnar epithelium (SCE) (with characteristic crypts and villi lined by mucus-secreting columnar cells and goblet cells), which is considered pathognomonic of Barrett's oesophagus. The similarity between SCE in Barrett's oesophagus and incomplete intestinal metaplasia in the stomach resulted in the use of methylene blue for selective staining of SCE. In a controlled pilot study Canto *et al.* showed methylene blue can selectively and reproducibly stain SCE in Barrett's oesophagus with high accuracy[11]. There are at least three other published studies from investigators in Germany[12] and the United States[13,14] that also demonstrated that methylene blue improves the detection of specialized columnar epithelium in Barrett's oesophagus. In particular, the diagnosis of short-segment Barrett's oesophagus is improved by methylene blue chromoendoscopy if the length of columnar epithelium is $>1 \,\text{cm}$[13]. The absence of definite positive staining in patients without a short length of columnar epithelium is helpful in excluding the presence of specialized Barrett's oesophagus. Methylene blue has also been used for improved detection of intestinal metaplasia in the gastric cardia[14].

Methylene blue staining involves application of a mucolytic, followed by dye, followed by washing off excess dye. Surface mucus must be removed to increase the uptake of dye into epithelial cells. This can be accomplished by spraying a mucolytic agent. The technique for methylene blue staining reported by Japanese endoscopists involves ingestion of a proteolytic enzyme solution (proteinase or Pronase) followed by methylene blue in a capsule. This technique was adapted by Fennerty et al. for use in the United States[8] by substituting 10% solution N-acetylcysteine for Pronase and 0.5% solution of methylene blue (available as 1% solution, American Reagent, Shirley, New York) for the capsule. Both reagents are sprayed on the mucosa with a washing catheter in sequence. Excess dye is then washed off with syringes. The endpoint of staining is somewhat subjective and is the most difficult part to learn. Positive staining is defined as the presence of blue-stained mucosa that persists despite vigorous water irrigation. The endpoint of staining is reached when the staining pattern and appearance of stained mucosa is stable and no further stain washes off. Staining adds an average of 5–7 min to the endoscopic procedure time. The cost of the reagents is under $9.

In Barrett's oesophagus, methylene blue staining may be either focal or diffuse (>75% of Barrett's mucosa stains blue)[16]. The majority of patients with long-segment (>6 cm) Barrett's oesophagus have diffuse staining because SCE comprises the majority of the columnar mucosa[10,16]. The pattern of methylene blue staining is important because dysplastic and malignant Barrett's oesophagus appears to behave differently from non-dysplastic epithelium[16]. Increasing grade of dysplasia is significantly associated with focal areas of decreased stain intensity and/or increased stain heterogeneity (i.e. increasing proportion of light blue or pink unstained mucosa compared to dark blue mucosa)[16]. Endoscopically inapparent high-grade dysplasia and adenocarcinomas in Barrett's oesophagus can be diagnosed by directed biopsy to the heterogeneously stained or light blue/unstained epithelium[16,17]. The mechanism for this difference in the staining characteristics of non-dysplastic and dysplastic Barrett's oesophagus is hypothetical, but is felt to be due to the difference in the morphology of these cells. Based on laser-induced confocal fluorescence work, we believe that methylene blue is absorbed or diffuses into the cytoplasm and goblet cells in Barrett's oesophagus. In non-dysplastic Barrett's oesophagus, there are characteristic goblet cells and mucus-containing columnar cells with an orderly arrangement of nuclei at the base. In contrast, highly dysplastic Barrett's oesophagus is characterized by loss of goblet cells, increase in nuclear size, and decrease in cytoplasm. Hence, less methylene blue dye is absorbed and this results in abnormal or decreased staining.

The accuracy and cost-effectiveness of methylene blue-directed biopsy for detecting intestinal metaplasia and dysplasia/cancer is significantly higher than four-quadrant, jumbo random biopsy in a randomized controlled sequential study[14].

There is much ongoing controversy regarding the accuracy and utility of methylene blue chromoendoscopy for Barrett's oesophagus. The majority of studies reporting favourable outcomes[10–14,16,18,19] have larger sample sizes and those with unfavourable outcomes are limited to much smaller studies[20–24]. Hence, one possible explanation for the variability in the results of various studies is the effect of experience and the learning curve for this relatively new technique. There is also variability in the technique and lack of training in chromoendoscopy in most gastrointestinal training programmes.

Future improvements in chromoendoscopy for Barrett's oesophagus include its combination of staining with high-magnification endoscopy[25], the use of combination stains (such as cresyl violet)[18,26], improved and standardized techniques, and improved accuracy that comes with training and experience.

Methylene blue staining has also been used to aid in the diagnosis of flat or non-polypoid colorectal cancers that may not be endoscopically apparent[27]. Furthermore, aberrant crypt foci, the earliest identifiable precursor lesion of adenomas and cancer, have been characterized and endoscopically diagnosed using methylene blue staining in the colon combined with magnification endoscopy[28].

Indigo carmine

Indigo carmine is derived from a blue plant dye (indigo) and a red colouring agent (carmine). Unlike vital stains, this deep blue stain is not absorbed by gastrointestinal epithelium. It pools in crevices between epithelial cells and highlights small or flat lesions and defines irregularities in mucosal architecture, particularly when used with high-magnification or high-resolution endoscopy.

Indigo carmine has been used in combination with high-magnification endoscopy to diagnose the villiform appearance of Barrett's oesophagus[29]. In the stomach, indigo carmine can diagnose small gastric cancers[30]. In the duodenum it has been used to evaluate villous atrophy in patients suspected of having malabsorption from coeliac disease or tropical sprue[31]. In the colon it has been used to study the surface appearance of colonic crypts and discriminate between hyperplastic polyps (which have a typical 'pit' pattern) and adenomatous polyps (which have a 'groove' or 'sulci' pattern)[32]. It can also aid in the diagnosis of minute, flat or depressed colorectal tumours[33–36].

Indigo carmine is commercially available in the United States in a vial (0.8%, American Reagent Laboratories, Shirley, New York). It is generally used as a 0.08% solution in the colon.

REACTIVE STAINS

Congo red

Congo red is a pH indicator that changes from red to dark blue or black in acidic conditions. It has been used to map acid-producing epithelium in the stomach or in ectopic sites. It can help with the evaluation of post-vagotomy patients[37]. It has been used primarily for screening for early gastric cancers and for detecting synchronous lesions, in combination with methylene blue (which stains gastric intestinal metaplasia)[9,38]. The early gastric cancer will usually be identified as a 'bleached' area of mucosa that did not stain with either Congo red or methylene blue. Synchronous gastric cancers are present in up to 9% of patients when this combination staining technique is used. Congo red can also aid in the detection of intestinal metaplasia of the stomach, which is accompanied by gastric atrophy and decreased or absent acid production.

The technique for staining with Congo red involves stimulation of acid production with 250 μg of pentagastrin given orally. Then, during endoscopy, 0.5% sodium bicarbonate solution is sprayed prior to a 0.3–0.5% Congo red solution. A positive reaction (black colour change) results within minutes that delineates acid-secreting areas (blue–black) from non-acid-secreting areas (red).

Phenol red

Like Congo red, phenol red is a pH indicator. It detects alkaline pH by a colour change from yellow to red. A promising useful clinical application of phenol red is the detection of *Helicobacter pylori* infection in the stomach. The urease produced by the bacterium catalyzes hydrolysis of urea to NH_3 and CO_2, which results in increased pH. Hence, *H. pylori* can be observed in red-stained mucosa. Investigators have used the endoscopic phenol red test to improve the diagnosis of *H. pylori*[39] and map its distribution in the stomach[40,41]. The reported sensitivity and specificity in 108 patients studied was 100% and 84.6%, respectively. This technique has also been recently used to clarify the role of the organism in gastric carcinogenesis[40]. A prospective study by Japanese investigators of 79 patients with ($n = 65$) and without ($n = 14$) gastric adenocarcinoma[39] showed good correlation of red-colour change with actual *H. pylori* infection. Indeed, 59 of 65 patients with gastric cancer showed *H. pylori* infection using this endoscopic test, particularly those with differentiated tumours. Hence, the endoscopic phenol red test may potentially help researchers investigate the association of *H. pylori* with other disease conditions.

The technique of the endoscopic phenol red test involves treatment with a potent acid-suppressive agent in all patients and application of a mucolytic agent, dimethylpolysiloxane, and an anticholinergic drug just before endoscopy[39]. Then, during endoscopy, a solution of 0.1% phenol red and 5% urea is sprayed evenly over the gastric mucosal surface. A positive test consists of a colour change from yellow to red, which indicates the presence of *H. pylori*. Areas of gastric intestinal metaplasia will not change colour to red.

ENDOSCOPIC TATTOO

India ink

India ink consists of suspended inert carbon particles in aqueous or non-aqueous stabilizers and diluents[40]. Injection of India ink with a sclerotherapy needle is used to permanently mark locations of lesions. This is possible because the ink remains in the gastrointestinal wall for long periods of time; perhaps for life. This allows for easy intraoperative localization of colonic lesions or endoscopic surveillance of colonic tumours, such as malignant polyps or large sessile adenomas removed by piecemeal polypectomy[43–45]. It has also been used to mark the proximal and distal extent of Barrett's oesophagus[46]. The latter indication is relatively a new and potentially useful one in the research setting. For example, India ink could mark the squamocolumnar junction for longitudinal follow-up of the length of Barrett's oesophagus and surveillance after mucosal ablation. The black tattoo reportedly persists at least 36 months[46].

The dilution and technique of India ink tattooing is highly variable. India ink is frequently used unsterilized; however, the preferred methods for tattooing involve sterilization by autoclaving or gas sterilization. One described technique involves dilution of commercial-grade India ink with an equal volume of water, followed by sterilization by standard autoclaving processing[47]. Alternatively, the ink can be diluted with sterile bacteriostatic water (ratio 5 parts ink to 2 parts water) and passed through a Travenol 5-μm pore-size filter into sterile 5-ml vials (to remove large particulate material) before being autoclaved for 40 min[44]. The opened India ink vials are sterile for 2 h while unopened ones can be used up to 6 months after preparation.

Prior to injection, the vial should be shaken well and the ink drawn up into a 3 or 5 ml syringe attached to a sclerotherapy needle. Injections of 0.1–0.5 ml should be made to create intramucosal or submucosal blebs just proximal and distal to the colonic lesion and on the other quadrants of the colonic wall nearby. Multiple injections are recommended.

Although India ink tattooing is generally considered safe over the long term[44], several reports have raised concern about the adverse effects associated with India ink tattooing. In a comprehensive review of colonic tattooing with India ink, Nizam et al.[45] found at least 447 cases reported in the literature, with only five reports of complications (risk of 0.22%). These include allergic reactions[48], fat necrosis and inflammatory pseudotumours[49], and colonic abscess and focal peritonitis[50].

Purified carbon

A new product called Spot (GI Supply, Camp Hill, Pennsylvannia) is now commercially available in the United States and is the only Federal Drug Administration (FDA)-approved drug for endoscopic tattoo. It is a sterile, biocompatible, non-pyrogenic suspension containing highly purified carbon particles.

Indocyanine green

Indocyanine green makes a persistent tattoo and does not cause secondary tissue inflammatory change, unlike India ink[42]. This dye has not been extensively studied for endoscopic tattooing but deserves further evaluation.

Methylene blue

Methylene blue has been used to tattoo the colon wall for localization of lesions during surgery. However, it appears to cause a significant tissue reaction and fibrinoid necrosis of vessel walls and does not persist as long as India ink. In a study evaluating the tissue injury of India ink and methylene blue as tattoo agents, the latter was not grossly visible 7 days after injection, unlike the former which lasted at least 7 weeks[51]. Hence, methylene blue is a poor tattoo agent compared to India ink.

CONCLUSION

Chromoendoscopy is widely available, low cost, technically simple, and highly accurate. It is a valuable technique for improving endoscopic visualization and diagnosis. Chromoendoscopy is an inexpensive, safe, accurate, simple endoscopic technique that is underutilized in gastrointestinal practice. Chromoendoscopy should be part of the armamentarium of all endoscopists.

References

1. Chisholm EM, Williams SR, Leung JW, Chung SC, Van Hasselt CA, Li AK. Lugol's iodine dye-enhanced endoscopy in patients with cancer of the oesophagus and head and neck. Eur J Surg Oncol. 1992;18:550–2.
2. Yokoyama A, Ohmori T, Makuuchi H et al. Successful screening for early oesophageal cancer in alcoholics using endoscopy and mucosa iodine staining [See comments]. Cancer. 1995; 76:928–34.
3. Okumura T, Aruga H, Inohara H et al. Endoscopic examination of the upper gastrointestinal tract for the presence of second primary cancers in head and neck cancer patients. Acta Otolaryngol Suppl. 1993;501:103–6.
4. Woolf GM, Riddell RH, Irvine EJ, Hunt RH. A study to examine agreement between endoscopy and histology for the diagnosis of columnar lined (Barrett's) oesophagus. Gastrointest Endosc. 1989;35:541–4.
5. Seitz J, Monges G, Navarro P, Giovannini M, Gauthier A. Endoscopic detection of dysplasia and early oesophageal cancer: results of a prospective study with toluidine blue staining in 100 tobacco and alcohol abusers. Gastroenterol Clin Biol. 1990;14:15–21.
6. Hix WR, Wilson WR. Toluidine blue staining of the oesophagus. A useful adjunct in the panendoscopic evaluation of patients with squamous cell carcinoma of the head and neck. Arch Otolaryngol Head Neck Surg. 1987;113:864–5.
7. Chobanian SJ, Cattau EL Jr, Winters C Jr et al. In vivo staining with toluidine blue as an adjunct to the endoscopic detection of Barrett's oesophagus. Gastrointest Endosc. 1987;33:99–101.
8. Fennerty MB, Sampliner RE, McGee DL, Hixson LJ, Garewal HS. Intestinal metaplasia of the stomach: identification by a selective mucosal staining technique [See comments]. Gastrointest Endosc. 1992;38:696–8.
9. Tatsuta M, Iishi H, Okuda S, Taniguchi H. Diagnosis of early gastric cancers in the upper part of the stomach by the endoscopic Congo red–methylene blue test. Endoscopy. 1984;16:131–4.
10. Giler S, Kadish U, Urca L. Use of tolonium chloride in the diagnosis of malignant gastric ulcers. Arch Surg. 1978;113(2):136–9.
11. Canto MI, Setrakian S, Petras RE, Blades E, Chak A, Sivak MV Jr. Methylene blue selectively stains intestinal metaplasia in Barrett's oesophagus. Gastrointest Endosc. 1996;44:1–7.
12. Kiesslich R, Hahn M, Herrmann G, Jung M. Screening for specialized columnar epithelium with methylene blue: chromoendoscopy in patients with Barrett's oesophagus and a normal control group. Gastrointest Endosc. 2001;53:47–52.
13. Sharma P, Topalovski M, Mayo MS, Weston AP. Methylene blue chromoendoscopy for detection of short-segment Barrett's oesophagus. Gastrointest Endosc. 2001;54:289–93.
14. Canto MI, Setrakian S, Willis J et al. Methylene blue-directed biopsies improve detection of intestinal metaplasia and dysplasia in Barrett's oesophagus. Gastrointest Endosc. 2000; 51:560–8.
15. Morales T, Bhattacharyya A, Camargo E, Johnson C, Sampliner R. Methylene blue staining for intestinal metaplasia of the gastric cardia with follow-up for dysplasia. Gastrointest Endosc. 1998;48:26–31.
16. Canto M, Setrakian S, Willis J, Petras R, Chak A, MV Sivak J. Methylene blue staining of dysplastic and nondysplastic Barrett's oesophagus: an in vivo and ex vivo study. Endoscopy. 2001;33:391–400.
17. Canto M, Wu TT, Montgomery E, Kaloo AN. Methylene blue staining predicts dysplasia in Barrett's oesophagus. Gastrointest Endosc. 1999;49(4):AB 49.

18. Sueoka N, Tabuchi M, Nishigaki H, Sakamoto C, Kobayashi M, Sasajima K. Magnification endoscopy with vital dye staining for detection of a minute focus of early adenocarcinoma in Barrett's oesophagus. Gastrointest Endosc. 2001;53:AB150 (abstract).
19. Weerth AD, Brand B, Fritscher-Ravens A et al. High resolution zoom endoscopy combined with vital staining for improved accurate detection of dysplasia in Barrett's mucosa – preliminary results from an ongoing study. Gastrointest Endosc. 2001;53(5):AB160 (abstract).
20. Dave U, Shousha S, Westaby D. Methylene blue staining: is it really useful in Barrett's oesophagus? Gastrointest Endosc. 2001;53:333–5.
21. Gangarosa LM, Halter S, Mertz H. Methylene blue staining and endoscopic ultrasound evaluation of Barrett's oesophagus with low-grade dysplasia. Dig Dis Sci. 2000;45:225–9.
22. Jobson B, Goenka P, Manalo G, Thomas E. Methylene blue staining for intestinal metaplasia in Barrett's esophagus – is it as good as we think? Gastrointest Endosc. 1999;49:AB 52.
23. Breyer HP, Maguilnik I, Barros SG. Methylene blue can disclose intestinal metaplasia in Barrett's esophagus? Gastrointest Endosc. 2000;51:abstract A116.
24. Wo J, Ray M, Mayfield-Stokes S et al. Comparison of methylene blue directed biopsies and conventional biopsies in the detection of intestinal metaplasia and dysplasia in Barrett's esophagus. Gastrointest Endosc. 2001;53(In press).
25. Canto MIF, Wu T-T, Kalloo AN. High magnification endoscopy with methylene blue chromoendoscopy for improved diagnosis of Barrett's esophagus and dysplasia. Gastrointest Endosc. 2001;53:abstract 4171 (AB140).
26. Tabuchi M, Sueoka N, Fujimori T. Videoendoscopy with vital double dye staining (crystal violet and methylene blue) for detection of a minute focus of early adenocarcinoma in Barrett's oesophagus:a case report. Gastrointest Endosc. 2001;54(3):385–8.
27. Kudo S, Kashida H, Nakajima T, Tamura S, Nakajo K. Endoscopic diagnosis and treatment of early colorectal cancer. World J Surg. 1997;21:694–701.
28. Takayama T, Katsuki S, Takahashi Y et al. Aberrant crypt foci of the colon as precursors of adenoma and cancer. N Engl J Med. 1998;339:1277–84.
29. Stevens PD, Lightdale CJ, Green PH, Siegel LM, Garcia-Carrasquillo RJ, Rotterdam H. Combined magnification endoscopy with chromoendoscopy for the evaluation of Barrett's esophagus. Gastrointest Endosc. 1994;40:747–9.
30. Ida K, Hashimoto Y, Takeda S, Murakami K, Kawai K. Endoscopic diagnosis of gastric cancer with dye scattering. Am J Gastroenterol. 1975;63:316–20.
31. Siegel LM, Stevens PD, Lightdale CJ et al. Combined magnification endoscopy with chromoendoscopy in the evaluation of patients with suspected malabsorption. Gastrointest Endosc. 1997;46:226–30.
32. Axelrad AM, Fleischer DE, Geller AJ et al. High-resolution chromoendoscopy for the diagnosis of diminutive colon polyps: implications for colon cancer screening. Gastroenterology. 1996;110:1253–8.
33. Jaramillo E, Watanabe M, Slezak P, Rubio C. Flat neoplastic lesions of the colon and rectum detected by high-resolution video endoscopy and chromoscopy. [See comments]. Gastrointest Endosc. 1995;42:114–22.
34. Iishi H, Kitamura S, Nakaizumi A et al. Clinicopathological features and endoscopic diagnosis of superficial early adenocarcinomas of the large intestine. Dig Dis Sci. 1993;38:1333–7.
35. Tada M, Katoh S, Kohli Y, Kawai K. On the dye spraying method in colonofiberscopy. Endoscopy. 1977:8:70–4.
36. Mitooka H, Fujimori T, Maeda S, Nagasako K. Minute flat depressed neoplastic lesions of the colon detected by contrast chromoscopy using an indigo carmine capsule. Gastrointest Endosc. 1995;41:453–9.
37. Donahue P, Bombeck C, Yoshida Y, Nyhus L. The simplified endoscopic congo red test for completeness of vagotomy. Surg Gynecol Obstet. 1986;163:287–9.
38. Tatsuta M, Okuda S, Taniguchi H. Diagnosis of minute cancers by the endoscopic Congo red–methylene blue test. Endoscopy 1983;15:252–6.
39. Azuma T, Kato T, Hirai M, Ito S, Kohli Y. Diagnosis of *Helicobacter pylori* infection. J Gastroenterol Hepatol. 1996;11:662–9.
40. Iseki K, Tatsuta M, Iishi H, Baba M, Ishiguro S. *Helicobacter pylori* infection in patients with early gastric cancer by the endoscopic phenol red test [Published erratum appears in Gut. 1998; 42:450]. Gut. 1998;42:20–3.

41. Boyanova L, Stancheva I, Todorov D et al. Comparison of three urease tests for detection of *Helicobacter pylori* in gastric biopsy specimens. Eur J Gastroenterol Hepatol. 1996;8:911–14.
42. Fennerty MB. Tissue staining. Gastrointest Endosc Clin N Am. 1994;4:297–311.
43. Botoman VA, Pietro M, Thirlby RC. Localization of colonic lesions with endoscopic tattoo. Dis Colon Rectum. 1994;37:775–6.
44. Shatz BA, Weinstock LB, Swanson PE, Thyssen EP. Long-term safety of India ink tattoos in the colon. Gastrointest Endosc. 1997;45:153–6.
45. Nizam R, Siddiqi N, Landas SK, Kaplan DS, Holtzapple PG. Colonic tattooing with India ink: benefits, risks, and alternatives. Am J Gastroenterol. 1996;91:1804–8.
46. Shaffer RT, Francis JM, Carrougher JG et al. India ink tattooing in the esophagus. Gastrointest Endosc. 1998;47:257–60.
47. Hyman N, Waye JD. Endoscopic four quadrant tattoo for the identification of colonic lesions at surgery. Gastrointest Endosc. 1991;37:56–8.
48. Gallo R, Parodi A, Cozzani E, Guarrera M. Allergic reaction to India ink in a black tattoo. Contact Dermatitis. 1998;38:346–7.
49. Coman E, Brandt LJ, Brenner S, Frank M, Sablay B, Bennett B. Fat necrosis and inflammatory pseudotumor due to endoscopic tattooing of the colon with india ink [See comments]. Gastrointest Endosc. 1991;37:65–8.
51. Park SI, Genta RS, Romeo DP, Weesner RE. Colonic abscess and focal peritonitis secondary to india ink tattooing of the colon [See comments]. Gastrointest Endosc. 1991;37:68–71.
52. Lane KL, Vallera R, Washington K, Gottfried MR. Endoscopic tattoo agents in the colon. Tissue responses and clinical implications. Am J Surg Pathol. 1996;20:1266–70.

21
CT- or MRI-based virtual colonography

A. G. SCHREYER and H. HERFARTH

THE PRESENT

Virtual endoscopy, otherwise virtual colonoscopy, represents a technique which basically depicts two-dimensional (2D) sectional images such as computerized tomography (CT) or magnetic resonance imaging (MRI) with computed three-dimensional (3D) models. These computed 3D models of hollow organs represent the actual hollow organ, i.e. the colon in a virtual world. Even virtual flights through these models or other visualization methods are possible. Vining[1] first described in 1996 a virtual flight through the colon. Meanwhile many other different applications and studies regarding this visualization technique have been done.

The application of CT- or MRI-based virtual colonography for the detection of polyps as a screening method is of major interest.

SENSITIVITY AND SPECIFICITY OF VIRTUAL COLONOGRAPHY

Several papers have addressed the sensitivity and specificity of virtual colonography in detecting polyps. Conventional colonoscopy, however, remains the reference for this new technique. Fenlon and co-workers[2] compare prospectively virtual CT colonography with conventional colonoscopy in 100 patients at high risk for colorectal neoplasia. Polyps ≥ 10 mm were detected with a sensitivity of 91%. Polyps ranging from 5 mm to 9 mm were visualized with 82% sensitivity, whereas small polyps smaller than 5 mm were seen with 55% sensitivity. These workers conclude that virtual and conventional colonoscopy had similar efficacy for the detection of polyps that were 6 mm or more in diameter (Table 1). Other studies have confirmed these sensitivity data[3]. Similar studies using MRI as the primary imaging method were performed by Pappalardo et al.[4] and Luboldt et al.[5], revealing a sensitivity above 90% for polyps ≥ 10 mm.

Table 1 Sensitivity of virtual colonography in comparison to conventional colonoscopy in 100 patients[2]

Polyp size	Total (n)	True positive (n)	False negative	False positive (n)	Sensitivity (%)
All	115	82	33	19	71
>10 mm	22	20	2	2	91
6–9 mm	40	33	7	8	82
1–5 mm	53	29	24	9	55

Table 2 Factors influencing the sensitivity and specificity of virtual CT- or MRI-based colonography

Bowel preparation
Learning curve
Experience of the centre in the development and sophistication of virtual CT and MR techniques
Technique: volume or surface rendering
Software
Bias (studies so far were exclusively done in patients with a history of polyps)

A certain problem for a widespread use is the fact that these studies were conducted by investigators in specialized departments which have certain experience. Pescatore et al.[6] described the sensitivity and specificity in polyp detection of two teams respectively composed of a radiologist and a gastroenterologist. In the first 24 patients both teams had a sensitivity of 100% and 92% with a specificity of 42% and 58%. After a re-evaluation of the results of these first 24 patients and learning sessions the sensitivity was decreased in subsequent 25 patients to 50% (both teams) with an increased specificity of 79% in each team.

Generally there are several potential reasons for varying sensitivities and specificities in this young technique. The quality of the 3D reconstruction depends on good bowel preparation, as in conventional endoscopy. Another reason for varying sensitivities can be the learning curve in performing this type of examination. Different visualization techniques such as volume- or surface rendering, and the quality of software packages, together with the performance of the hardware, could also influence the outcome (Table 2).

PATIENT COMPLIANCE

Another problem for virtual colonography as a screening method is patient compliance. Probably the statement of Silvermann bears a lot of truth: 'Currently virtual colonography needs the same bowel preparation as conventional colonoscopy, which is for a majority of the patients the most annoying part of the colonoscopy procedure'[7]. Therefore, if there is a suspicion of polyps in the colon the polyp should be removed on the same day using conventional colonoscopy, because the bowel is already prepared.

THE FUTURE

There are many ongoing efforts and studies concerning improvements in virtual endoscopy. First some other potential applications of virtual endoscopy of the gastrointestinal (GI) tract should be discussed.

OTHER VIRTUAL MODALITIES IN THE GI TRACT

The colon seems to be the most suitable part of the GI tract for virtual endoscopy. It has a clear structure and can be contrasted very easily. There are some studies performing virtual endoscopy of the stomach. However, virtual gastroscopy is difficult to perform because most of the pathological changes are within the mucosa, which cannot be depicted adequately using sectional imaging methods. Consequently most studies are feasibility studies with no major clinical impact.

Virtual endoscopy of small bowel represents an interesting application depicting fistulas or inflammatory changes, especially in patients with Crohn's disease. A study performed by our group[8] demonstrated the feasibility of this technique in patients with inflammatory bowel disease (Table 3).

POTENTIAL IMPROVEMENTS TO INCREASE SENSITIVITY AND SPECIFICITY

There are several technical solutions to improve the sensitivity and specificity of virtual colonoscopy: one approach involves different 3D rendering methods, which could improve the efficiency in diagnosis. For example 'virtual pathology' can be a method to depict the whole bowel wall within one comprehensive image. Virtual pathology represents a computer algorithm which basically cuts the colon like a pathologist and opens and flattens the intraluminal wall mathematically. So all bowel folds, together with potential pathological changes, can be analysed within one projection.

Another tool to improve the diagnostic outcome is computer-assisted diagnosis. This technique consists of computer algorithms which analyse the surface of a hollow organ wall for irregularities[9]. Then the software highlights the suspicious areas on 3D and 2D images. Consequently the radiologist can double-check these areas manually.

Table 3 Quality of virtual endoscopy of the small bowel in 30 patients with inflammatory bowel disease

Quality of the small bowel virtual endoscopy (%)	
Total	($n = 30$) 100
Poor	10
Fair	60
Good	30

CT- OR MRI-BASED VIRTUAL COLONOGRAPHY

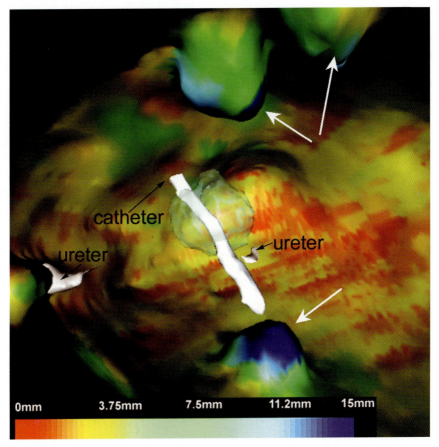

Figure 1 Virtual cystoscopy: the colour indicates the wall thickness of the hollow organ – blue means thickened wall – the three white arrows indicate the tumour[10]

A more straightforward approach for computer-assisted diagnosis could be the colour-coding of wall thickness in virtual endoscopy[10]. Using this technique a colour scale ranging from red to blue represents the thickness of a wall within the 3D model (Figure 1). This colour adds depth information to virtual endoscopy, which indicates even subtle wall changes. All these techniques together could certainly improve the sensitivity of virtual endoscopy.

IMPROVING PATIENTS' COMPLIANCE

Certainly the need for bowel preparation as in conventional colonoscopy is one of the major drawbacks in patient compliance concerning the virtual system. Various solutions have been experimented with in order to avoid this bowel preparation. Currently the common approach for CT and MR imaging without bowel cleansing represents the so-called 'fecal labeling' technique[11]. For CT imaging the preparation consists of a high-density contrast medium (e.g. barium), which is added to each meal. After bowel scanning the remaining highly contrasted faeces can be subtracted digitally, resulting in a so-called 'electronic cleansing'. In MR imaging similar techniques ranging from adding positive contrast media gadolinium[11] to negative contrast media such as barium (which appears as a low signal in MR imaging in contrast to CT) are under evaluation[12]. There are still no studies addressing the sensitivity or specificity of faecal labelled examination to detect pathological changes of the bowel.

To conclude, there are still many dramatic technical changes in CT- or MR-based virtual colonoscopy. Even the modalities and rendering techniques to depict the bowel lumen are subject to change. For example, virtual pathology with computer-assisted diagnostic tools or an unprepared and faecal labelled bowel could be potential new approaches in this fascinating and still-evolving technique.

References

1. Vining DJ. Virtual endoscopy: is it reality? Radiology. 1996;200:30–1.
2. Fenlon HM, Nunes DP, Schroy PC 3rd, Barish MA, Clarke PD, Ferrucci JT. A comparison of virtual and conventional colonoscopy for the detection of colorectal polyps. N Engl J Med. 1999;341:1496–503.
3. Rex DK, Vining D, Kopecky KK. An initial experience with screening for colon polyps using spiral CT with and without CT colography (virtual colonoscopy). Gastrointest Endosc. 1999;50:309–13.
4. Pappalardo G, Polettini E, Frattaroli FM et al. Magnetic resonance colonography versus conventional colonoscopy for the detection of colonic endoluminal lesions. Gastroenterology. 2000;119:300–4.
5. Luboldt W, Bauerfeind P, Wildermuth S, Marincek B, Fried M, Debatin JF. Colonic masses: detection with MR colonography. Radiology. 2000;216:383–8.
6. Pescatore P, Glucker T, Delarive J et al. Diagnostic accuracy and interobserver agreement of CT colonography (virtual colonoscopy). Gut. 2000;47:126–30.
7. Bauerfeind P, Luboldt W, Debatin JF. Virtual colonography. Baillieres Best Pract Res Clin Gastroenterol. 1999;13:59–65.
8. Schreyer AG, Herfarth HH, Albrich H et al. MR-based virtual endoscopy of the small intestine and colon in patients with inflammatory bowel disease. Gastroenterology. 2000;118:A886 (abstract).
9. Summers RM, Selbie WS, Malley JD et al. Polypoid lesions of airways: early experience with computer-assisted detection by using virtual bronchoscopy and surface curvature. Radiology. 1998; 208:331–7.
10. Schreyer AG, Fielding JR, Warfield SK et al. Virtual CT cystoscopy: color mapping of bladder wall thickness. Invest Radiol. 2000;35:331–4.
11. Weishaupt D, Patak MA, Froehlich J, Ruehm SG, Debatin JF. Faecal tagging to avoid colonic cleansing before MRI colonography. Lancet. 1999;354:835–6.
12. Lauenstein T, Holtmann G, Schoenfelder D, Bosk S, Ruehm SG, Debatin JF. MR colonography without colonic cleansing: a new strategy to improve patient acceptance. Am J Roentgenol. 2001;177:823–7.

22
Three-dimensional endoscopy

T. THORMÄHLEN, H. BROSZIO and P. N. MEIER

INTRODUCTION

Diagnosis and intervention in endoscopy is based on image sequences of a video camera. But an image sequence provides no depth information. If the usual stereoscopic human sight is missing, navigation of instruments is difficult. Recognition and evaluation of pathological structures and the estimation of their spatial extension can be achieved only by experience. Diagnosis is very subjective. Measurement of calibrated data for colour and texture and a three-dimensional (3D) reconstruction of pathological structures can make endoscopic diagnosis more objective and reproducible. Therefore this chapter presents an approach that allows 3D reconstruction from endoscopic image sequences.

The described approach estimates the camera motion and uses the estimated camera motion to reconstruct the 3D scene. The camera motion must be estimated from the image sequence because it cannot be controlled or accurately measured. In computer vision this problem is called the *structure from motion* problem. Since the structure from motion approach only requires an image sequence as input data an ordinary flexible monocular video endoscope can be used without any modifications.

In most known approaches which generate an endoscopic 3D scene a special endoscope is developed or an additional device is inserted into the working channel of the endoscope. Schubert and Müller[1] presented a structured light method for bronchoscopy which can be used for measurement of hollow biological organs. The 3D scene is estimated by the deformation of a projected ring of laser light. A laser fibre probe is inserted into the instrument channel. Armbruster and Scheffler[2] developed a prototype of an endoscope that measures the 3D scene by deformation of several projected lines. The accuracy of this structured light method is increased by a phase shift of the lines. Kemper et al.[3] have examined the deformation of a 3D scene with an electronic-speckle-pattern interferometer. A stiff minimal inversive endoscope is extended with an external holographic camera. Some endoscope manufacturers offer special stereo endoscopes for 3D reconstruction or 3D visualization. Since stereo endoscopes have two optical channels they have a larger diameter than usual endoscopes and are not often used in practice.

Other approaches exist that only evaluate the endoscopic image sequence to reconstruct the 3D scene. Yeung et al.[4] proposed a shape from shading algorithm. Deguchi et al.[5] have used a structure from motion approach for endoscopic image sequences, where camera motion and 3D scene is estimated by the factorization method.

The approach presented here consists of two parts. First the very robust estimation of camera motion. Based on conventional feature point detection and correspondence analysis, the robustness of the estimation is achieved by using a highly efficient outlier detection of misaligned correspondences. The second part consists in the reconstruction of the 3D scene by using the known camera motion.

The next section describes the proposed estimation algorithm for the motion of the camera. The following sections explain the reconstruction of the 3D scene, and give some results. The chapter ends with conclusions.

ROBUST ESTIMATION OF CAMERA MOTION

The estimation method illustrated in Figure 1 consists of three processing steps: detection of feature points, determination of correspondences and robust estimation of the camera motion parameters.

Detection of feature points

The feature points are detected with subpixel accuracy using the Harris feature point detector[6]. For each image of the sequence a list of feature point coordinates

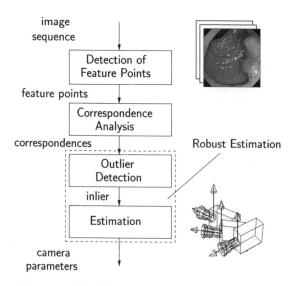

Figure 1 Steps of the proposed algorithm to estimate camera motion parameters

$L = \{\mathbf{p}_1, \ldots, \mathbf{p}_i, \ldots, \mathbf{p}_M\}$ is extracted, where $\mathbf{p}_i = (x_i, y_i)^\top$ is the image coordinate of a feature point.

Correspondence analysis

The feature points in list L and L' of two successive images are assigned by measuring normalized cross-correlation between 15×15 windows surrounding the feature points. The correspondences are established for those feature points which have the highest cross-correlation. This results in a list of correspondences $L_c = \{q_1, \ldots, q_i, \ldots, q_N\}$, where $q_i = (\mathbf{p}_i, \mathbf{p}'_i)$ is a correspondence.

Estimation of camera translation

For the estimation of camera motion parameters from corresponding feature points, the real camera must be represented by a mathematical camera model. Required relation between corresponding feature points in two images follows from the motion model.

Camera model

The perspective camera model with the focal length f describes the projection of a 3D scene coordinate $\mathbf{P} = (X, Y, Z)^\top$ into the image plane (Figure 2). The projected 2D image point $\mathbf{p} = (x, y)^\top$ can be calculated as follows

$$\mathbf{p} = \begin{pmatrix} x \\ y \end{pmatrix} = \frac{f}{Z} \cdot \begin{pmatrix} X \\ Y \end{pmatrix} \qquad (1)$$

A shift of the optical centre and the third-order radial lens distortions with respect to the image centre (barrel and cushion) are also taken into account. For simplification these camera parameters are mentioned only briefly. A detailed camera model can be found in ref. 7.

Motion model

The proposed algorithm to estimate the translation of the camera and the scene geometry is based on a motion model, which is illustrated in Figure 3. The general camera operation is given by the position of the camera centre $\mathbf{C}' = (C_X, C_Y, C_Z)^\top$ relative to the coordinate frame (X, Y, Z) and the rotation matrix $\mathbf{R}$, which can be

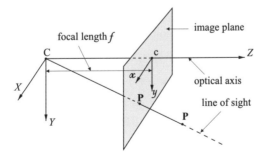

Figure 2 Camera model

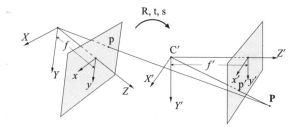

Figure 3 Projection of 3D point **P** for a moved camera

specified as three successive rotations $\mathbf{R}_\varphi$, $\mathbf{R}_\vartheta$ and $\mathbf{R}_\rho$ around the Y-, X- and Z-axes, respectively. The rotations are named throughout this paper as φ for pan, ϑ for tilt and ρ for roll.

If **P** is a 3D point represented in the camera coordinate frame (X, Y, Z) and **P**′ represents the same point in the coordinate frame (X', Y', Z') after the camera operation, then the transformation is given by

$$\mathbf{P}' = \mathbf{R}(\mathbf{P} - \mathbf{C}') \qquad (2)$$

with

$$\mathbf{R} = \mathbf{R}_\rho \mathbf{R}_\vartheta \mathbf{R}_\varphi$$

$$= \begin{bmatrix} \cos\rho & \sin\rho & 0 \\ -\sin\rho & \cos\rho & 0 \\ 0 & 0 & 1 \end{bmatrix} \begin{bmatrix} 1 & 0 & 0 \\ 0 & \cos\vartheta & \sin\vartheta \\ 0 & -\sin\vartheta & \cos\vartheta \end{bmatrix} \begin{bmatrix} \cos\varphi & 0 & -\sin\varphi \\ 0 & 1 & 0 \\ \sin\varphi & 0 & \cos\varphi \end{bmatrix}$$

$$= \begin{bmatrix} r_{11} & r_{12} & r_{13} \\ r_{21} & r_{22} & r_{23} \\ r_{31} & r_{32} & r_{33} \end{bmatrix} \qquad (3)$$

It is convenient not to make the camera translation explicit, and instead to represent the transformation in equation (2) with

$$\mathbf{t} = (t_X, t_Y, t_Z)^\top = -\mathbf{R}\,\mathbf{C}' \qquad (4)$$

Equation (2) can be rewritten as

$$\mathbf{P}' = \mathbf{R}\mathbf{P} + \mathbf{t} \qquad (5)$$

Combining equations (1) and (5) the relationship between the image coordinates $\mathbf{p}_i = (x_i, y_i)^\top$ and $\mathbf{p}'_i = (x'_i, y'_i)^\top$ of a projected 3D point $\mathbf{P}_i = (X_i, Y_i, Z_i)^\top$

can be expressed as

$$x'_i = f' \frac{r_{11}x_i + r_{12}y_i + r_{13}f + f(t_X/Z_i)}{r_{31}x_i + r_{32}y_i + r_{33}f + f(t_Z/Z_i)}$$
$$y'_i = f' \frac{r_{21}x_i + r_{22}y_i + r_{23}f + f(t_Y/Z_i)}{r_{31}x_i + r_{32}y_i + r_{33}f + f(t_Z/Z_i)}$$
(6)

where the focal length after the camera operation is $f' = sf$.

Assuming pure translation and the absence of zoom, which is valid for most endoscopic image sequences, the motion model can ignore rotation and zoom operations. Therefore equation (6) can be simplified

$$x'_i = \frac{x_i + f(t_X/Z_i)}{1 + (t_Z/Z_i)}$$
$$y'_i = \frac{y_i + f(t_Y/Z_i)}{1 + (t_Z/Z_i)}$$
(7)

Elimination of Z_i between these two equations gives

$$(y'_i - y_i)\frac{t_X}{t_Z} - (x'_i - x_i)\frac{t_Y}{t_Z} + \frac{x'_i y_i - x_i y'_i}{f} = 0 \qquad (8)$$

With the substitution

$$\frac{t_X}{t_Z} = \tilde{t}_X \qquad \frac{t_Y}{t_{YZ}} = \tilde{t}_Y \qquad (9)$$

and two correspondences the following linear equation system can be built

$$\begin{bmatrix} (y'_1 - y_1) & (x_1 - x'_1) \\ (y'_2 - y_2) & (x_2 - x'_2) \end{bmatrix} \begin{pmatrix} \tilde{t}_X \\ \tilde{t}_Y \end{pmatrix} = \begin{pmatrix} (x_1 y'_1 - x'_1 y_1)/f \\ (x_2 y'_2 - x'_2 y_2)/f \end{pmatrix} \qquad (10)$$

This equation system can be solved explicitly for $\tilde{t}_X$ and $\tilde{t}_Y$.

The translation of the camera can be determined only up to an arbitrary scale factor k, which leads into the following constraint

$$\sqrt{t_X^2 + t_Y^2 + t_Z^2} = k \qquad (11)$$

This constraint implies the third motion parameter t_Z with

$$t_Z = \frac{k}{\sqrt{\tilde{t}_X^2 + \tilde{t}_Y^2 + 1}} \qquad (12)$$

Outlier detection

Due to misalignments, usually some of the correspondences are incorrect. To achieve a robust estimation of camera motion parameters, a random sampling algorithm[8] for outlier detection is employed. Two correspondences are sufficient to calculate the camera motion parameters using equations (10) and (12). Because equation (10) can be solved explicitly this calculation is very fast. Support of this parameter set is measured by evaluating how good the displacements of the other correspondences can be expressed by this parameter set. If it does not match the majority of the correspondences, a new parameter set is chosen randomly until a satisfying solution is found. The correspondences, which support the satisfying solution are called inliers – the others outliers. Only the inliers are applied to estimate the camera motion parameters and 3D scene in the following processing step.

Estimation of camera motion

The camera motion parameters are estimated using a least-squares technique applied to all inlier correspondences by minimizing the residual error of the cost function (13) over $\tilde{t}_X$ and $\tilde{t}_Y$.

$$\sum_i \epsilon_i(\tilde{t}_X, \tilde{t}_Y)^2 \to \min \qquad (13)$$

with the residuals

$$\epsilon_i(\tilde{t}_X, \tilde{t}_Y) = (y'_i - y_i)\tilde{t}_X - (x'_i - x_i)\tilde{t}_Y + (x'_i y_i - x_i y'_i)/f \qquad (14)$$

The minimum of the cost function can be calculated by linear regression.

3D RECONSTRUCTION

The scheme for automatic reconstruction of the 3D scene from an image sequence is illustrated in Figure 4. The reconstruction process consists of three steps:

1. Calculation of 3D coordinates for each detected inlier feature point giving a cloud of 3D feature points.
2. Generation of a 2D triangle mesh in the image plane with inlier corners as vertices, which converts the 3D point cloud into a triangle surface description.
3. Final texturing to assign a natural look to the 3D reconstruction.

Calculation of 3D coordinates

Known camera motion enables the calculation of 3D point coordinates belonging to each inlier correspondence. The triangulation of two lines of sight from two different cameras gives the 3D coordinate for each correspondence. Due to erroneous detection of feature points the lines of sight do not intersect in most cases (Figure 5).

Therefore, a correspondence of two 3D points $\tilde{\mathbf{P}}_i$ and $\tilde{\mathbf{P}}'_i$ can be determined for each feature point separately. The 3D points are located where the lines of sight

THREE-DIMENSIONAL ENDOSCOPY

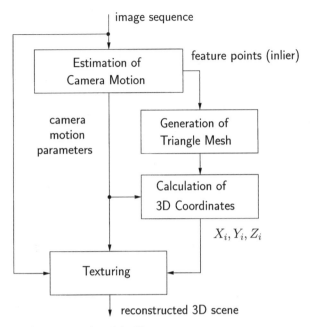

Figure 4 Scheme for reconstruction of the 3D scene

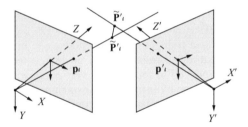

Figure 5 Triangulation of lines of sight for correspondences

have their smallest distance. The arithmetic mean of $\tilde{\mathbf{P}}_i$ and $\tilde{\mathbf{P}}'_i$ gives final 3D coordinate $\mathbf{P}_i$.

Generation of a triangle mesh

The shape representation of the 3D reconstruction by a textured triangle mesh is common practice. For recovering the shape, the cloud of 3D points has to be converted into a triangle mesh. Diverse possibilities to triangulate a 3D point cloud make the recovering of the shape problematic. Therefore, an approach is used to triangulate the feature points in the image plane by using Delaunay triangulation[9]. Depending on the 2D triangle meshes in the image planes the 3D points are connected to a 3D triangle mesh (Figure 6).

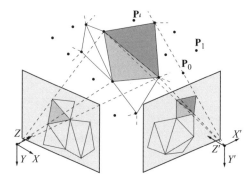

Figure 6 Generation of 2D triangle meshes in the image planes. Connecting 3D points advised by the 2D triangle meshes

The characteristics of the Delaunay triangulation and the known correspondences of feature points between successive images enables the generation of a closed and coherent 3D triangle mesh. The feature points of each image of sequence belonging to inlier correspondences, provide a partition of the 3D triangle mesh.

Texturing

For a realistic-looking 3D model a texturing algorithm is used, which estimates the texture for each surface triangle from the endoscopic image sequence. The principle of binding texture information from an image sequence to a single surface triangle was introduced in ref. 10. The vertices of a surface triangle are projected into the image plane by using the known camera parameters. The projected triangle contains the image part which defines the texture map. Due to many possibilities of images from which the texture information can be taken, each triangle is assigned to that image of the sequence which ensures the highest texture resolution defined by the ratio of texture elements per surface area.

RESULTS

This method has been applied to an image sequence that was recorded on a real intervention. In the image sequence a polyp in the colon can be seen (Figure 7). Figure 8 shows the result of feature point detection for the first two images of the sequence. The feature points detector finds 930 feature points in the first image and 898 in the second. With this feature point set 528 correspondences are calculated (Figure 9). From these the applied random-sampling algorithm selects 348 supported correspondences (Figure 10), that are used to estimate camera motion. With the estimated camera motion a 3D reconstruction of the polyp is performed. Figure 11 exhibits the reconstructed 3D scene from two different views.

THREE-DIMENSIONAL ENDOSCOPY

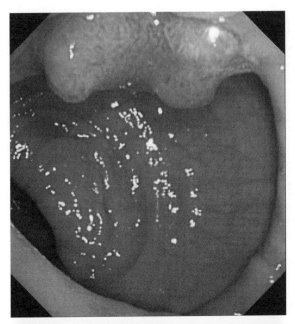

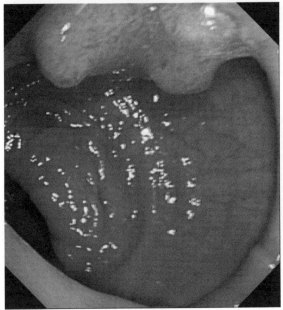

Figure 7 First two images of the sequence 'polyp in colon'

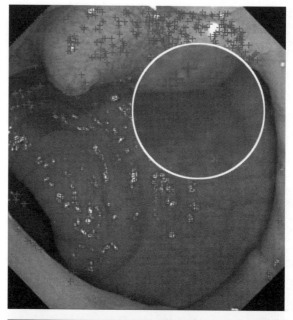
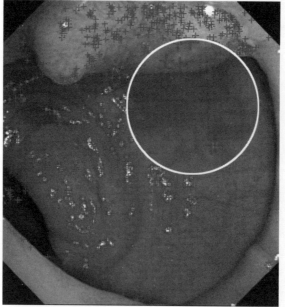

Figure 8 Extracted feature points from the first two images of the sequence

THREE-DIMENSIONAL ENDOSCOPY

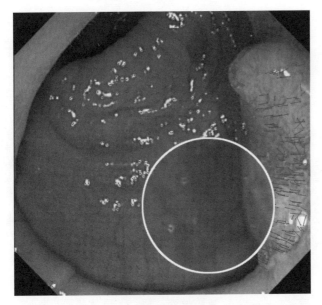

Figure 9 Displacement vectors of corresponding corners between the first two images

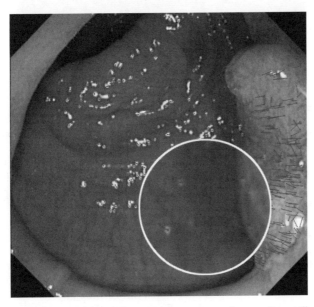

Figure 10 Displacement vectors of the remaining correspondences after outlier elimination (inlier = green displacement, outlier = blue displacement)

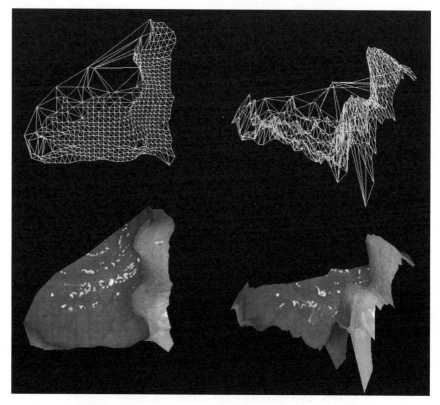

Figure 11 Reconstructed 3D surface model 'polyp in colon' from two different views with and without textures

CONCLUSIONS

A robust estimation technique for computation of camera translation was presented. Based on conventional feature detection and correspondence analysis the robustness of the approach is achieved by the use of a highly efficient outlier detection of misaligned correspondences. The camera translation estimator is based on a very fast linear regression technique that computes accurate parameters.

These accurate parameters are used to reconstruct the observed 3D scene. Though the reconstruction method is still very basic the potential of the approach is obvious. In future work the accuracy of the method should be improved and the estimation error should be analyzed.

Visualization of the reconstructed 3D scene offers new possibilities for diagnosis and intervention planning. Furthermore it will be possible to visualize a virtual endoscope in the 3D scene, which informs the physician about the current position of the endoscope. This 3D representation of an operation can support navigation or can help to teach medical students in an illustrative manner.

References

1. Schubert M, Müller A. Evaluation of endoscopic images for 3-dimensional measurement of hollow organs. Biomed Eng. 1998;43:32–3.
2. Armbruster K, Scheffler M. Messendes 3D-Endoskop. Horizonte. 1998;12:15–16.
3. Kemper B, Merker A, Lai A, von Bally G. A novel electronic-speckle-pattern interferometer (ESPI) for dynamic holographic endoscopy. Fifth International Conference on Optics Within Life Sciences, Vol. V: Optics and Lasers in Biomedicine and Culture. 1998; Heraklion, Crete, Greece; Springer, 1999.
4. Yeung SY, Tsui HT, Yim A. Global shape from shading for an endoscope image. Medical image and computer assisted intervention. Second International Conference Proceedings MICCAI'99, 1999, pp. 328–32.
5. Deguchi K, Sasano T, Arai H, Yoshikawa H. 3-D shape reconstruction from endoscope image sequences by the factorization method. IEICE Trans Inform Syst. 1996;E79-D(9):1329–36.
6. Harris C, Stephens M. A combined corner and edge detector. Proceedings of 4th Alvey Vision Conference. 1988;11:147–51.
7. Tsai RY. A versatile camera calibration technique for high-accuracy 3-D machine vision metrology using off-the-shelf cameras and lenses. IEEE Trans Robot Automat. 1987;3:000–00.
8. Fischler MA, Bolles RC. Random sample consensus: a paradigm for model fitting with application to image analysis and automated cartography. Commun Assoc Comput Machinery. 1981;24:381–95.
9. Lischinski D. Incremental Delaunay triangulation. In: Heckbert PS, ed. Graphics Gems IV. New York: Academic Press, 1994:43–59.
10. Niem W, Broszio H. Mapping texture from multiple camera views onto 3D-object models for computer animation. International Workshop on Stereoscopic and Three-Dimensional Imaging. Santorini, Greece; 6–8 September 1995.

Section VIII
New endoscopic equipment – new visual perspectives?

23
Wireless capsule endoscopy

A. GLUKHOVSKY and H. JACOB

INTRODUCTION

Attempts at minimal invasive examination of the body lumens were first made in ancient times. Hippocrates (5th century BC) described the use of a primitive anoscope (speculum) for examination of haemorrhoids[1]. In 1806 a sophisticated external illumination source was introduced by Philip Bozzini, thereby improving the ability to introduce an optical instrument into the gastrointestinal tract[2]. Introduction of the technique of air insufflation by George Kelling in 1901[2] enabled physicians to increase the field of view by expanding the lumen, which is usually in a collapsed state. One of the major technological advances in the development of the endoscope was the invention of the flexible fibreoptic gastroscope by Harold Hopkins in 1951[3]. Dr Basil Hirshowitz was the first physician to clinically use this instrument in late 1960s[4]. Further technological improvements paved the way for a variety of different types of endoscopes enabling both diagnosis and therapy of the oesophagus, stomach, proximal small intestine, and colon.

Another technology, unrelated to endoscopy, emerged in the late 1950s. This was based on the invention of the transistor and subsequent miniaturization of electronic devices. Based on miniaturization technology, and on encapsulation technologies, autonomous swallowable wireless telemetric devices appeared. Various devices introduced the ability to measure temperature[5], pressure[6] and pH[7] within the gastrointestinal tract.

The end of the 20th century was characterized by numerous technological breakthroughs, including the availability of high-quality CMOS (complementary metal oxide semiconductors) imagers[8], miniature LEDs (light-emitting diodes) emitting white light[9], and miniature low-power UHF (ultra-high-frequency) band transmitters/controllers based on advances in mixed signal ASIC (application specific integrated circuit) technology.

These technological breakthroughs enabled the merger of the two branches of development, resulting in a new, revolutionary type of endoscopy – wireless capsule endoscopy, developed and tested in trials by Given Imaging Ltd[10].

Following the first healthy volunteer human trial conducted in 1999[10], the first clinical trial was performed subsequently in 2000[11]. The diagnostic yield of the new device was studied in a series of animal[12] and human clinical trials[13].

As a new technology it is referred to by numerous names in the literature, usually emphasizing one of its features, e.g.: wireless capsule endoscope, capsule endoscope, swallowable video capsule, video capsule, and video pill. For the sake of clarity we suggest using either the term wireless capsule endoscope or capsule endoscope when referring to this new device.

MATERIALS AND METHODS

Evaluation of performance of the wireless endoscope was performed using the Given Imaging Diagnostic System. The system includes the M2A™ wireless capsule endoscope, the wearable DataRecorder™ for wireless reception of data and storage of the acquired images, and the Rapid™ workstation for presentation and analysis of the acquired images.

The M2A™ wireless capsule endoscope is shown in Figure 1a. A schematic appears in Figure 1b. The wireless capsule endoscope has a cylindrical shape,

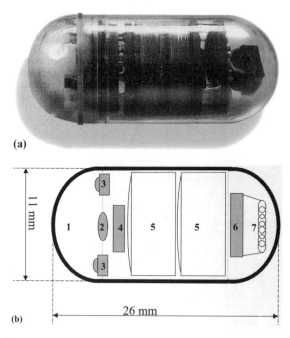

Figure 1 Wireless capsule endoscope: (**a**) external view; (**b**) schematic cross-section: 1, optical dome; 2, short focal aspheric lens; 3, white LEDs; 4, CMOS imager; 5, batteries; 6, ASIC transmitter; 7, antenna

diameter 11 mm, and length 26 mm. It has two convex domes, one of them being the optical dome (1). The intestine is illuminated through the optical dome by white LEDs (3). The obtained image is focused by a short focal aspherical lens (2) on the CMOS imager (4). The optical dome has a shape that prevents the light reflected by the dome itself reaching the imager, thus degrading image quality. The capsule is powered by two standard watch batteries (5). An ASIC transmitter (6) is located in the rear dome. The radiofrequency (RF) signal is transmitted by the antenna (7).

After ingestion of the capsule the patient is free to return to his/her routine daily activity. The capsule acquires and transmits images of the intestine for approximately 8 h. During this period the transmitted images and data are received by a sensor array attached to the patient's abdomen. The images and data are recorded and stored by a DataRecorder worn by the patient on a special belt.

After approximately 8 h the patient returns the DataRecorder to the clinic. The images and the data stored in the DataRecorder are transferred to the workstation, where the Rapid software is used for presentation and analysis.

The wireless capsule endoscope is disposable, and is naturally excreted from the body.

RESULTS

To evaluate the use of the wireless capsule endoscope on humans, more than 270 healthy volunteers and patients ingested the M2A capsule in clinical trials.

Between December 1998 and March 2001, 73 healthy volunteers ingested the M2A capsule. In each of these cases the volunteers easily swallowed the capsule, it moved smoothly through the gastrointestinal tract, and the volunteers excreted the capsule naturally without any adverse events.

To further evaluate the safety and efficacy of the wireless capsule endoscope, two feasibility trials were completed in Israel. Between September 2000 and early March 2001, 35 patients ingested the M2A capsule for these studies. The resulting information either confirmed or expanded the suspected diagnosis in 22 of the 35 patients, or 63%. The patients ingested the capsule smoothly with no adverse events in all of these cases.

Another clinical trial was performed in the United States between October 2000 and January 2001[13]. Twenty patients were examined in the trial, and underwent a capsule endoscopy and push enteroscopy. The trial was designed to evaluate the ingestion, passage, and excretion of the M2A capsule, assess the diagnostic ability of the wireless capsule endoscopy in comparison to push enteroscopy, obtain subjective assessments from patients comparing the wireless capsule endoscopy and the push enteroscopy procedures, and analyse retrieved capsules for integrity during passage through the digestive tract.

The results of the trial were as follows.

Easy ingestion and safe passage

The M2A capsule was easily ingested, passed safely through the digestive tract and was naturally excreted without causing complications or reported discomfort.

Improved diagnostic yield

The Given Imaging Diagnostic System detected new findings in the small intestine not previously detected by other methods, such as endoscopy and barium X-rays. In the clinical trial the wireless capsule endoscope detected physical abnormalities in 12 of 20 patients, or 60%, while push enteroscopy detected physical abnormalities in seven of 20 patients, or 35%. In total, 14 lesions were detected in 13 of 20 patients participating in the clinical trials using either the Given System, push enteroscopy or surgical techniques. The wireless capsule endoscopy detected 12 of the 14 lesions, or 86%, while push enteroscopy detected seven of 14 lesions, or 50%[13]. Samples of images acquired in the clinical trials are presented in Figure 2.

Clear preference for the Given system

The subjective assessments of patients showed a definite preference for the capsule endoscopy procedure over push enteroscopy.

No deterioration during passage

Although the M2A capsule is designed to be disposable, the clinical trial protocol required retrieval of the capsules after use in order to prove the integrity of

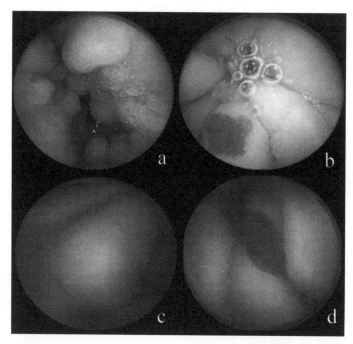

Figure 2 Examples of images acquired by capsule endoscope from the small intestine. **(a)** Brunner's gland hyperplasia; **(b)** multiple telangiectasia on gastric fold; **(c)** small bowel carcinoid tumour; **(d)** active duodenal bleeding

the M2A capsule during passage through the gastrointestinal tract. All of the retrieved capsules were intact and showed no signs of deterioration.

Between January 2001 and June 2001 an additional 127 patients ingested the M2A in 10 different clinical trial sites in Europe. The preliminary data from these trials confirmed the prior data regarding performance of the M2A wireless endoscope.

Careful analysis of the images acquired by the capsule endoscope reveals striking anatomical details. Detailed images of the arterial and venous structures are seen. Linear (usually radial) white structures are seen regularly (Figure 3). These may represent the lymphatic infrastructure of the small bowel. The lymphatics are seen coursing perpendicular to villi, which are clearly visualized. When followed, the lymphatics can be seen running along the veins. Careful analysis of abnormal capsule endoscopy reveals a new dimension of pathological features, many of which may be related to the normal anatomical features noted above. In order to provide an explanation of the observed findings the bio-optical principles governing image acquisition of the capsule were reviewed. A number of these principles derived from the design of the optical head – such as illumination efficiency, viewing geometry, and the special optical dome, in our opinion are playing an important role. In addition, physiological image acquisition seems to be playing an important role in obtaining the detailed information visualized by the capsule.

DISCUSSION

With the accumulation of increasing amounts of clinical data it is emerging that, while there is obvious similarity between push endoscopy ('wired endoscopy') and wireless capsule endoscopy, there are also differences, especially in the mode of image acquisition. The wireless endoscope is not just an endoscope without wires.

Below we hypothesize regarding the unique combination of physiological, physical, and optical reasons that may be producing the observed differences between the two endoscopic approaches. Some of the concepts suggested in this chapter will require further experimental verification.

Capsule endoscopy enables exploration of the gastrointestinal tract in its natural physiological state. This physiological endoscopic inspection yields detailed images of the small bowel as presented above. Several physiological and bio-optical principles may be playing a role in the capsule's ability to acquire these highly detailed images:

1. Exploration of the gastrointestinal tract in its physiological state (physiological image acquisition):
    (a) no use of air insufflation,
    (b) no insertion of bundles of cables,
    (c) natural propulsion by peristalsis,
    (d) use of liquid in gastrointestinal tract as an optical window.
2. Use of the special optical dome resulting in:
    (a) improved illumination efficiency,
    (b) more effective geometry of the field of view.

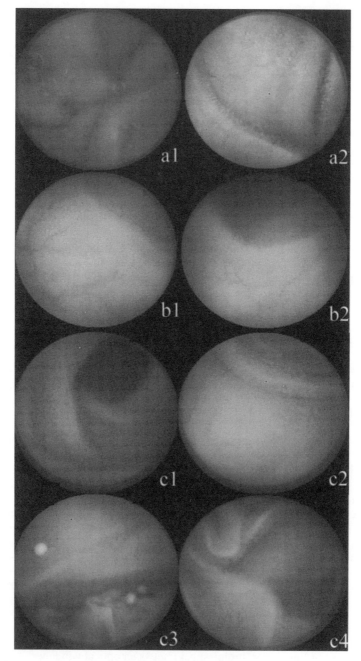

Figure 3 Anatomical details. **(a1, a2)** normal villi appearance; **(b1, b2)** normal vascular structures; **(c1, c2, c3, c4)** normal lymphatics

Geometrical and optical differences between the image acquisition in wired and wireless endoscopy are described below.

The simplified schematic diagram in Figure 4 describes geometrical interrelationships for the push enterosope inserted in the intestine (a) for the capsule endoscope (b). Figure 4a shows the tip of the endoscope (1). The endoscope includes an illumination source (2), and lens (3), producing a field of illumination (4), and field of view (5) respectively. Collapse of the intestinal wall (6) may obscure either field of view or field of illumination. This technological problem is solved in push enteroscopy by insufflating the intestine with air (7), which results in pushing the intestinal walls from the tip of the endoscope.

Figure 4b shows the wireless capsule endoscope (1) in the intestine. The capsule includes its illumination sources (2), and the lens (3), comprising field of illumination (4), and field of view (5) respectively. In order to prevent collapse of the intestinal wall (6), and obscuring either the field of illumination or the field of view especially, a specially designed optical dome (8) covers both the illumination and the lens. The space remaining between the dome and the intestinal wall may be occupied by liquid (or sometimes a mixture of liquid and air bubbles).

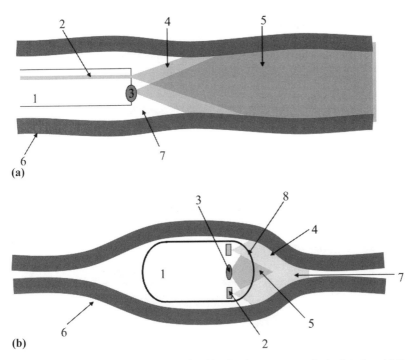

Figure 4 Geometrical and optical interrelationships for the enteroscope in the intestine. (**a**) Push enteroscope: 1, endoscope inside the intestine; 2, illumination source; 3, lens; 4, field of illumination; 5, field of view; 6, intestinal wall; 7, air filling, due to insufflation. (**b**) Capsule endoscope: 1, wireless capsule endoscope inside the intestine; 2, illumination source; 3, lens; 4, field of illumination; 5, field of view; 6, intestinal wall; 7, liquid filling, intestinal liquids; 8, optical dome

The field of view of most of the commercially available enteroscopes is within the range 120–140°, similar to the capsule endoscope.

It has been observed in multiple experiments that, while the intestine is full of air during push enteroscopy, in the case of capsule endoscopy it is filled with liquid, with occasional air bubbles and air pockets.

Although air insufflation solves problems of optical obstruction, it also changes the normal physiological condition of the intestine. The possible physiological and physical results of airless endoscopy are discussed below.

1. Physical and optical aspects of capsule endoscopy:
   (a) The illumination efficiency is higher due to the fact that the illumination angle is not sharp, and most of the illumination is efficient and is returned by the object back to the camera. Figure 5a shows that the illumination is not being returned in the case of air insufflation. Figure 5b demonstrates that in the case of airless endoscopy illumination is more effective.
   (b) Under normal physiological conditions, intestinal contents, after several hours of fasting, are evacuated from the small intestine. Under these conditions the intestine is collapsed and most of the remaining space is filled with the liquid, sometimes mixed with air bubbles of various sizes. Application of insufflation fills the intestine with air, leaving the liquid spread only on the intestinal wall – in the form of a thin layer of moisture. Therefore viewing conditions during airless endoscopy are similar to underwater viewing. Insufflation alters these conditions. With air insufflation the villi collapse, while they are floating freely in the

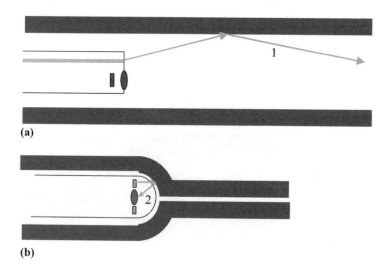

Figure 5 Efficiency of illumination in air insufflating and airless endoscopy. (**a**) In the air insufflating case the illumination is less efficient due to the fact that some of the rays are reaching the intestine at flat edges, and are not returned back to the lens and to the camera. (**b**) In the airless endoscopy most of the illumination is returned back to the lens due to sharp edges of illumination, close to perpendicular

liquid in the absence of insufflation. Villi that are floating are more visible when examined endoscopically.

Excellent visualization of villi may present an alternative explanation to the appearance of white lines in the acquired image. As was suggested earlier, these lines may be associated with lymphatic structures. However, Figure 6 shows that lines of different colour may be observed along folds of the intestinal wall (5), as compared to the colour observed in the alternative direction (6, 7).

2. Physiological aspects: in addition to the difference in the geometry and physics of image acquisition, physiological changes may develop due to insufflation and increasing air pressure in the intestine:
   (a) Under normal pysiological conditions blood pressure in the blood vessels of the gastrointestinal tract may be within the following range: arterioles 40–80 mmHg, capillaries 20–40 mmHg, and venules 15–30 mmHg. During push enteroscopy the pressure may reach above 300 mmHg[14], significantly higher than blood pressure. We may speculate that this increase in pressure may decrease blood flow to small vessels, and in some cases even temporarily arrest the flow. Although we have not found reference to the tamponade effect in enteroscopy, this phenomenon has been well known in laparoscopy for more than a century[2]. In rare cases air insufflation may even cause a fatal air embolism during gastrointestinal endoscopy[14].
   (b) Insufflation of the small intestine, and insertion of long flexible tube, affects the pressure receptors embedded in the small intestinal wall. We

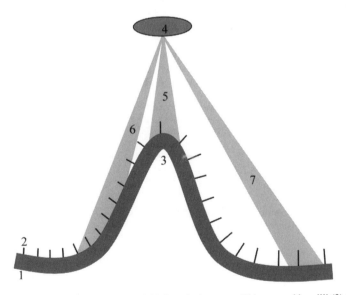

Figure 6 Schematic drawing of mucosal fold. Intestinal mucosa (1) is covered by villi (2). The area of mucosal fold is marked shown (3). The camera (4) is examining the intestinal wall. While looking at the fold, most of the visible area will belong to mucosa (5). Viewing at other directions (6, 7) will usually result in more villous cover

may speculate therefore that, unlike in the case of wireless endoscopy, the intestine is not being seen in physiological, 'natural', conditions.
(c) Examination of the intestine under physiological conditions enables measuring of additional physiological parameters, some of them unrelated to the image, e.g. gastric emptying, small and large bowel passage times.

SUMMARY

The clinical study report concluded that wireless capsule endoscopy is able to acquire satisfactory images and to identify pathologies in the small intestine that are not accessible by push enteroscopy or other methods. The clinical study report also stated that the wireless capsule endoscopy procedure is simple, low-risk and less traumatic than other procedures, that the procedure is more convenient for both the patient and the physician, and that it may be used in a variety of settings.

The study also suggests that wireless capsule endoscopy has advantages over conventional wired endoscopy due to its ability to perform examination of the gastrointestinal tract under normal physiological conditions.

References

1. Adams F (trans). The Genuine Works of Hippocrates. London: Sydenham Society, 1849:820–1.
2. Litynski GS. The History of Laparoscopy. Frankfurt/M: Bernert Verlag, 1996.
3. Hopkins HH, Kapany NS. A flexible fiberscope, using static scanning. Nature. 1954;173:39–41.
4. Hirshowitz BE. A fiberoptic flexible esophagoscope. Lancet. 1963;2:388.
5. Zworykin VK. Radio pill. Nature. 1957;179:898.
6. Mackay RS. Endoradiosonde. Nature. 1957;179:1239–40.
7. Noller HG. Die Endoradiosonde. Zur elektronischen pH-Messung im Magen und ihre klinische Bedeutung. Dtsche Med Wochenschr. 1960;85:1707.
8. Fossum ER. Active pixel sensor: Are CCD's dinosaurs?, Proc SPIE. 1993;1900:2–14.
9. Craford MG, Holonyak N, Frederick AK. In pursuit of the ultimate lamp. Sci Am. February 2001:49–53.
10. Iddan G, Meron G, Glukhovsky A, Swain P. Wireless capsule endoscopy. Nature. 2000;405:417.
11. Appleyard M, Glukhovsky A, Swain P. Wireless-capsule diagnostic endoscopy for recurrent small-bowel bleeding. N Engl J Med. 2001;344:232–3.
12. Appleyard M, Fireman Z, Glukhovsky A et al. A randomized trial comparing wireless capsule endoscopy with push enteroscopy for the detection of small-bowel lesions. Gastroenterology. 2000;199:1431–8.
13. Lewis B, Swain P. Capsule endoscopy in the evaluation of patients with suspected small intestinal bleeding, a blinded analysis: the results of the first clinical trial. Gastrointest Endosc. 2001;53:AB70.
14. Katzgraber F, Glenewinkel F, Fischler S. Mechanism of fatal air embolism after gastrointestinal endoscopy. Int J Legal Med. 1998;111:154–6.

24
When is enteroscopy useful?

G. GAY

Enteroscopy will be useful for the management of small bowel disease in a patient if it facilitates an accurate diagnosis. It will be even more useful if, in addition, it offers a therapeutic possibility.

In this context its role will be considered as really useful when the oesogastroduodenoscopy is limited to lesions situated before the second part of the duodenum, and the ileocolonoscopy suggests a diagnostic procedure within 70 cm of the ileum by the anal route, and before the angle of Treitz by the oral route.

In the past, surgical endoscopy was the only method. It is still the only endoscopic exam which allows complete exploration of the small intestine. Its rate of morbidity is not negligible. Its application is complex and it needs good cooperation between surgeon and endoscopist. In the past few years there has been a development of non-surgical enteroscopy with a video push enteroscope (VPE). With this endoscope (length 2.79 m), it is possible to explore all of the jejunum and, with an overtube, the first loops of the ileum. Diagnostic and therapeutic procedures are possible. In comparison with other radiological/morphological methods we can say the VPE is useful in obscure, chronic, overt and/or occult bleeding; suspicion of enteropathy; follow-up of familial adenomatosis polyposis; and in patients with Peutz–Jegher's syndrome. Its usefulness is more anedoctal when the small intestine is affected by systemic diseases, infectious diseases (AIDS), drug damage or in follow-up of transplantations. However, progress is permanent; on the one hand, improvement in endoscopy can be applied to VPE – for example variable stiffness and flexibility endoscope; on the other hand, entero-CT scan and entero-MRI are available, and recently the first results of a Given Imaging® capsule in four chronic bleeding patients were published. In these conditions comparative evaluations are mandatory; but VPE will nevertheless be the only method which facilitates both biopsies and therapeutic procedures.

25
Focal point: oesophago-cardial transition

H. W. BOYCE

If minimal air insufflation of the proximal and mid-oesophagus is utilized during endoscopy, the closed lower oesophageal sphincter region may be readily demonstrated. At the point of closure of the proximal end of the sphincter, several (usually four to six) longitudinal symmetrical mucosal folds can be seen to disappear in the centre of the closed lumen. This closure point produces a rosette appearance with the lumen being precisely centred at the point where these longitudinal folds converge. The rosette closure site represents the proximal margin of the lower oesophageal sphincter (LOS). The tone of the LOS relaxes with primary or secondary peristalsis and also opens in response to gentle insufflation. As the closed normal oesophageal sphincter is approached with the endoscope it will relax with gentle scope pressure, and with passage through the sphincter there is little or no detectable resistance. As the high-pressure sphincter zone relaxes, one can identify the normal location of the squamocolumnar mucosal junction 1.5–2 cm beyond. This mucosal junction corresponds to the distal margin of the LOS.

The squamous mucosa of the oesophagus is pink-grey in colour and contrasts sharply with the orange-red or salmon colour of the gastric columnar epithelium. The oesophageal squamous mucosa is only slightly transparent and reflects light moderately while the columnar epithelium is relatively opaque.

With minimal inflation the junction of the squamous or columnar epithelium appears at or less than 2 cm above the hiatus as a slightly irregular or undulating line, the so-called ora serrata or 'Z' line. With continued inflation pressure, especially when a hiatal hernia is present, this irregular mucosal junction becomes straighter and loses its serrated contour. This mucosal junction is located at the distal or caudad margin of the LOS segment at or just below the oesophageal diaphragmatic hiatus. This line of demarcation between the two types of mucosa is readily identifiable in the absence of pathological changes. If there is uncertainty about the location of this mucosal junction it can be dramatically demonstrated by application of several millilitres of Lugol's iodine solution through an endoscopic catheter around its circumference[1]. This will promptly stain the glycogen in the oesophageal squamous mucosa a brown–black colour. In addition to surface characteristics and colour the normal distal extent of the oesophageal squamous epithelium is also clearly demarcated by the level of abrupt disappearance of multiple, linear, frequently branching, small blood vessels that disappear at the proximal margin of the gastric folds of the cardia along the junction of squamous and columnar epithelium[2].

After the endoscope is passed into the proximal stomach a retroversion manoeuvre should be performed to view the cardia and fundus. In the normal setting the insertion tube of the endoscope can be seen coming through a short intra-abdominal segment of the oesophagus. The LOS closure in this region is sustained throughout respiration and during moderate insufflation of the stomach, except that transient relaxation in response to primary or secondary peristalsis can be observed. The angle of His on the greater curvature aspect, being closely approximated to the normal squamocolumnar junction, is another landmark for the oesophagogastric muscular junction. This area is also called the submerged or abdominal segment of the oesophagus[3].

When a hiatal hernia is present, several linear gastric folds normally are seen in the cardia[1,4,5]. These folds normally terminate at the level of the normal location of the squamocolumnar mucosal junction. Therefore, this termination point of the folds can be utilized endoscopically and radiographically as a marker for the approximate normal location of the normal squamocolumnar mucosal junction. The cephalad margins of the longitudinal gastric folds also correspond to the level of the oesophagogastric muscular junction. The proximal margins of these folds, combined with the distal extent of the linear oesophageal vessels, provide the best endoscopic landmark for the muscular junction between oesophagus and stomach, and as a marker for the expected normal location of the squamocolumnar mucosal junction. These relationships to the oesophagogastric muscular junction can also be demonstrated on surgical and autopsy specimens.

The level of the squamocolumnar mucosal junction, the level of disappearance of the linear oesophageal vessels, and the proximal extent of the gastric mucosal folds are anatomical features that can be utilized in the precise endoscopic diagnosis of hiatal hernia and reflux sequelae, including the columnar-lined or Barrett's oesophagus. They will also be helpful in placement of sutures, clips or intramural injections being developed as endoscopic antireflux procedures.

References

1. Boyce HW. Endoscopic definitions of esophagogastric junction regional anatomy. Gastrointest Endosc. 2000;51:586–92.
2. De Carvalho CAF. Sur l'angio-architecture veineuse de la zone de transition oesophagogastrique et son interpretation fonctionnelle. Acta Anat. 1966;64:125–62.
3. Hill LD, Kozarek RA, Kraemer SJM et al. The gastroesophageal flap valve: in vitro and in vivo observations. Gastrointest Endosc. 1997;336:924–32.
4. McClave SA, Boyce HW, Gottfried MR. Early diagnosis of columnar-lined oesophagus: a new endoscopic diagnostic criterion. Gastrointest Endosc. 1987;33:413–16.
5. Boyce HW. Hiatus hernia and peptic diseases of the oesophagus. In: Sivak MV, editor. Gastroenterologic Endoscopy, 2nd edn. Philadelphia: WB Saunders, 2000:580–97.

Index

acetic acid 144–5
acute pancreatitis 91
Adamek, H E 36, 90–3
adenocarcinoma 55
   Barrett's oesophagus 173
   LIFS 176
   PDT 59
   phenol red stain 189
adenoma 59, 69, 158, 164, 169
adenomatous polyps 100–1, 103
adenomyomatosis 154
agent detection imaging (ADI) 134
AIDS 225
air insufflation 215, 222–4, 226
Albert, J 90–3
alosetron 9
American Society for Gastrointestinal Endoscopy (ASGE) 112, 123
5-aminolevulinic acid (5-ALA) 59, 61, 174–6, 178–9
anal canal 5–6
anatomical resection 143
angiography 42, 43
animal models 109
anorectal brain network 6–7, 9
Armbruster, K 199
arterial (chemo) embolization 143–4
autofluorescence 61–2, 174, 179
Aziz, Q 4

Bar-Meir, S 109–11
Barish, M A 94–106
barium 98, 198
Barrett's oesophagus 227
   adenocarcinoma 173
   chromoendoscopy 183, 186–8, 189–90
   early cancer detection 56, 59, 66
   fluorescence endoscopy 178, 179

LIFE-GI 62
LIFS 176
OCT 64
Becker, T 69–75
Bektas, H 69–75
Bhutani, M S 47
bile duct
   carcinoma 42, 155–6
   stones 41–2, 48, 91, 152
   ultrasound 155–6
biliary disease, ultrasound 151–7
biliary strictures 91
biliary tree 41–2, 91
Binmoeller, K F 37
biofeedback training 9
biopsy 167–8
   chromoendoscopy 187
   minilaparoscopy 13–14, 16, 19
   PDT 59
bleeding, scintigraphy/PET 79–80
Blomley, M J K 132–9
blood pool imaging 81–2
Bolondi, L 127–31
Börner, A R 79–89
Boyce, H W 226–7
Bozzini, P. 215
BR14 134
brain mapping 3–12
brainstem 6–8
Breer, H 90–3
bronchoscopy 199
Broszio, H 199–211

Calhoun, P 97
camera model 201
camera motion estimation 204, 206
camera translation estimation 201–4, 210
Canto, M I F 182–93

INDEX

carmine dye staining   59
Catalano, M F   45
Celli, N   127–31
cerebellum   6–8
Choi, D   133
cholangiocarcinoma   42, 155–6
cholangiocellular carcinoma (CCC)   71–2
cholangiography, intraoperative   41
cholangitis   91
   infectious   155
   primary sclerosing   71, 91, 155
cholecystectomy   21, 48
cholecystitis   154
cholecystolithiasis   152, 153
choledochal cysts   91
choledocholithiasis   90, 152–3
cholestatic liver disease   151
cholesterol polyps   154
chromoendoscopy   56–9, 60, 66, 182–93
chronic pancreatitis   33–9
   EUS   44–8
   MRCP   91
cingulate gyrus   6–8
cirrhosis   17–19, 160
   HCC   71, 84, 164
   lesions or nodules   164–9
   microbubbles   135
   resection   70, 71
   ultrasound   127–31
coenzymes   174
colitis   178
   see also ulcerative colitis
colon
   cancer   55, 102–3
   chromoendoscopy   188
   cleansing   98, 100
   laparoscopy and endoscopy   27
   MRI   92
   polyps   98, 99, 100–2, 206–10
colonoscopy   53, 92, 195
   cf virtual colonography   194
   simulators   109, 110
colorectal cancer   55, 66, 92, 147
   cirrhosis   164
   PET   85–6
   virtual colonoscopy   97–103
colorectal neoplasia
   CT colonography   101
   virtual colonography   194
columnar epithelium   186, 226
computer-assisted diagnosis   196–7
computer-based simulators   110–11
computerized tomography (CT)
   3D imaging   95–6
   colorectal cancer   85–6
   entero-CT scan   225
   gallbladder   152
   gastro-oesophageal cancer   84

jaundice   151
liver metastases   72
liver tumours   73, 74, 161–4
multi-headed   40–1
pancreatic cancer   42–4, 48
portal venous phase   158
scan acquisition   98–9
spiral   43, 72, 162
computerized tomography (CT) colonography   97–103
computerized tomography (CT)-based virtual colonography   194–8
confocal laser microscopy   65
congo red   184, 186, 188–9
contrast staining   182, 185, 188
contrast ultrasound sonography   163–4
conventional B-mode imaging (CBM)   134
correspondence analysis   201, 206, 210
cortical imaging   3–12
Cosgrove, D O   132–9
Cothren, R M   177
cresyl violet   188
Crohn's disease   196
crypts of Lieberkühn   62
CTAP   168

Dachman, A H   101
Definity   132
Deguchi, K   200
Delauney triangulation   206
Delvaux, M   112–24
Devière, J   33–9
diffuse liver disease
   microbubbles   134–6
   ultrasound   127–31
Digital Imaging and Communication in Medicine (DICOM)   121, 122, 123
DSA   168
Dumonceau, J-M   33–9
duodenum, chromoendoscopy   188
dye spraying   56–9, 62
dye staining   27
dysplasia
   see also high-grade dysplasia
   adenocarcinoma   173
   chromoendoscopy   183, 187
   early detection   66
   fluorescent endoscopy   176, 178–9
   low-grade   173, 176
   optical biopsy   65
dysplasia-associated lesion or mass (DALM)   56, 60
dysplastic gastric adenoma   59

EASIE   109
echo pattern   128
Edmundowicz, S A   41
Eker, C   177

INDEX

electronic cleansing 198
Enck, P 3–12
Endlicher, E 173–81
endogastric lesions, laparoscopy and endoscopy 27
endogenous tissue autofluorescence 174
endoscopic retrograde cholangiopancreatography (ERCP) 41, 42, 46, 72, 91–2
  cholangiocarcinoma 155
  cholangitis 155
  gallbladder 152
  PSC 155
  simulators 109, 110
endoscopic tattooing 182, 185, 189–90
endoscopic ultrasound (EUS) 40–9, 56, 66
  gallbladder 152
  miniprobes 65
  OCT comparison 64
endoscopic ultrasound (EUS)-guided FNA 40, 41
endoscopically assisted wedge resection (EAWR) 23, 25, 27–8
endoscopically laparoscopic-assisted segmental resection (EASR) 24, 27–8
endoscopically laparoscopic-assisted transluminal resection (EATR) 24, 26, 27–8
endoscopy
  chromoendoscopy 56–9, 60, 66, 182–93
  chronic pancreatitis 33–9
  fluorescence 173–81
  history 215
  and laparoscopy 21–9
  LIFE 174, 176–9
  Minimal Standard Terminology 112–24
  reasons for 113–15
  simulators 109–11
  three-dimensional 199–211
  time for training 53–4
  video 53
  virtual 100
  wireless capsule 215–24, 225
  zoom 56, 62–4
endosonography, diagnostic advantages 40–9
endotherapy 33–8
Enlarger EndoTrainer 109
entero-CT scan 225
entero-MRI scan 225
enteroscopy, when is it useful 225
epiphrenic diverticula 27
epithelium
  columnar 186, 226
  metastases 158
  squamous 226–7
Erlangen models 109–10
European Society for Gastrointestinal Endoscopy (ESGE) 112, 123
evoked potentials, cortical 3–4

exogenous fluorophores 174–6
extracorporeal shockwave lithotripsy (ESWL) 34, 36
extrahepatic tumours 71–2

faecal labelling technique 198
faecal tagging 100
feature points detection 200–1, 206, 210
Fenlon, H M 101, 102, 194
Fennerty, M B 187
Feussner, H 21–9
fibrosis 17–18, 19
Fletcher, J G 98, 99, 101
fluorescence endoscopy 173–81
(F-18)fluorodeoxyglucose (FDG) PET 83–6
focal liver lesions 133–4, 158–60
focal nodular hyperplasia (FNH) 17
  diagnostic approach 158, 164, 166, 169
  microbubbles 133, 134
  preoperative imaging 69, 73
  scintigraphy/PET 82–3
Fong, Y 147
Fornari, F 163
10-French stent 36
Frericks, H S B 69–75
Frieling, T 3
functional magnetic resonance imaging (fMRI) 4–5, 6, 9

Gaiani, S 127–31
Galanski, M 69–75
gallbladder
  cancer 154
  polyps 154
  ultrasound 152–4
gallstones 152
GASTER project 119, 120
gastric columnar epithelium 226
gastro-oesophageal cancer, PET 84
Gay, G 225
Gerken, G 13–20
GI-Mentor 110–11
Given Imaging Ltd 215, 216, 218, 225
glucagon 98
Glukhovsky, A 215–24
Gossner, L 179
Gratz, K F 79–89

haemangiomas 69, 72–3, 82
  diagnostic approach 158, 165, 166
  microbubbles 134
Hara, A K 99, 103
Haringsma, J 179
Harris feature point detector 200
Harvey, C J 132–9
Harvey, R T 151
Hastier, P 47
Hawes, R H 40–9

INDEX

Helicobacter pylori 189
hepatic adenoma 73
hepatic space-occupying lesions,
    scintigraphy/PET 81–3
hepatobiliary scintigraphy 82
hepatocellular carcinoma (HCC) 17, 140–6,
    158, 162–3, 168
  cirrhosis 71, 84, 164
  microbubbles 133, 134
  preoperative imaging 71, 73
  scintigraphy/PET 82–3, 84
hepatolithiasis 91
Herfarth, H 194–8
hiatal hernia 226, 227
high-grade dysplasia
  early detection 55–6
  LIFS 176
  Lugol's solution 183
  PDT 59
  ulcerative colitis 173
hilar cholangiocarcinoma *see* Klatskin's tumour
Hinninghofen, H 3–12
hippocampus 6
Hippocrates 215
Hirshowitz, B. 215
Hollerbach, S 55–68
Hopkins, H 215
Huibregtse, 36

Immersion Medical 110
incomplete colonoscopy 102
India ink 185, 189–90
indigo carmine 185, 188
indocyanine green 190
insular cortex 6–8
International Working Group 45–6
intraductal ultrasound (IDUS) 42, 155–6
iris shutter phenomenon 73
irritable bowel syndrome 9

Jacob, H 215–24
jaundice 71–2, 151–2

Kapadia, C R 177
Kelling, G 215
Kemper, B 199
Klatskin's tumour 72, 155
Klempnauer, J 69–75
Knapp, W H 79–89
Kudo, S 62

laparoscopically assisted endoscopic resection
    (LAER) 23, 24, 25, 27–8
laparoscopy 13, 14
  and endoscopy 21–9
  mini 13–20
  video 22
laser-induced confocal fluorescence 187

laser-induced fluorescence spectroscopy (LIFS)
    174, 176, 177, 179
late-phase PIM 134
Lau, H 143
Laugier, R 37
Lees, W R 45
Legmann, P 43
Lehman, G A 53–4
Lehner, F 69–75
Levovist 132, 134
LIFE-GI system 62
light-induced fluorescence (LIF) 61–2, 66
light-scattering spectroscopy 65
light/laser-induced fluorescence endoscopy
    (LIFE) 174, 176–9
Lim, A K P 132–9
limbic circuitary 6–7
lipolytic activity 47
liver
  cell adenoma 69
  diffuse disease 127–31, 134–6
  metastases *see* metastases
  microbubbles 132–9
  minilaparoscopy 13–19
  morphology 127
  tumours
    benign 69, 72–3
    interventional therapy 140–50
    preoperative imaging 69–75
    unclear 158–70
  ultrasound 127–31
Livraghi, T 140–50
low-grade dysplasia
  LIFS 176
  ulcerative colitis 173
lower oesophageal sphincter (LOS)
    226, 227
Luboldt, W 194
Lück, R 69–75
Lugol's iodine solution 57, 183–4, 186,
    226–7

M2A^{TM} 63, 216–19
Macari, M 100
magnetic resonance cholangiopancreatography
    (MRCP) 72, 90–2
magnetic resonance colonography 92
magnetic resonance imaging (MRI) 168
  3D imaging 95
  as endoscopy substitute 90–3
  entero-MRI scan 225
  functional 4–5, 6, 9
  liver tumours 161
  resolution limits 40–1
  virtual endoscopy 100
magnetic resonance imaging (MRI)-based
    virtual colonography 194–8
magnetic resonance tomography 73, 74

INDEX

magnetoencephalography (MEG)   4, 5, 6, 7
main pancreatic duct (MPD)
   drainage   33–9
   stones   34–6, 37
   strictures   34, 36–7
manometry   81
Maratka, Z   113
maximum-intensity projection (MIP)
   83–4, 96
Meier, P N   199–211
Messmann, H   173–81
metastases
   liver   86, 146–8, 158, 163
      microbubbles   133–6
      MPR   96
      preoperative imaging   69, 72
methylene blue   56–8, 184, 186–8, 190
microbubbles   132–9
Miller, W T Jr   151
minilaparoscopy   13–20
Minimal Standard Terminology (MST)   46, 112–24
Mitake, M   42
Morrin, M M   102
motion model   201–3
motor evoked potential recording   9
Mukai, H   42
Müller, A   199
multi-planar reformation (MPR)   95–6

Nashan, B   69–75
Natterman, C   45
neoplastic polyps   154
neuroendocrine tumours   86–8, 133
Nicholson, F B   102
Nizam, R   190

α-fetoprotein (AFP)   164, 167, 168
occlusive carcinoma   102
oesogastroduodenoscopy   225
oesophageal cancers
   Lugol's solution   183
   toluidine blue   186
oesophageal dysfunction, scintigraphy/PET   80–1
oesophageal squamous cell carcinoma   55
oesophageal squamous mucosa   226–7
oesophago-cardial transition   226–7
oesophagus
   cortical imaging   4–5, 9
   laparoscopy and endoscopy   27
   submerged segment   227
Ohara, H   34–5
optical biopsy   65
optical coherence tomography (OCT)   64–5, 66
ora serrata   226
orbitoparietal cortex   6–8

orthotopic liver transplantation (OLT)   141, 142, 146
outlier detection   203–4, 210

PACS   95
pancreatic cancer   42–4, 48, 84–5, 91
pancreatic duct   91
   main   33–9
pancreatitis
   acute   91
   chronic   33–9, 44–8, 91
   MRCP   91
pancreatography   45
   see also endoscopic retrograde cholangiopancreatography (ERCP)
   MRCP   72, 90–2
Panjehpour, M   176, 177
Pappalardo, G   100, 194
parenchymal hyperpressure   33
parieto-orbital cortex (POC)   6–8
partial resection, liver   142–3, 146–8
patient compliance   195–6, 197–8
percutaneous ablation techniques   144–5, 148
percutaneous ethanol injection (PEI)   144–6, 148
percutaneous ultrasonography   90–1
peripheral cholangiocarcinoma   155
peritoneum, minilaparoscopy   13, 14, 15
perspective camera model   201
Pescatore, P   101, 195
Peutz–Jegher's syndrome   225
phase inversion mode (PIM), microbubbles   134
phenol red   185, 189
photodynamic diagnosis (PDT)   59–61
Piscaglia, F   127–31
'pit pattern' classification   62
polyps   92
   adenomatous   100–1, 103
   chromoendoscopy   188
   colon   98, 99, 100–2, 206–10
   CT colonography   100–1, 103
   gallbladder   154
   virtual colonography   194–5
Ponchon, T   37
porcelain gallbladder   154
portal hypertension   14, 128–9
portal thrombosis   141, 142, 167
positron emission tomography (PET)   9, 168
   intestinal sensory functions   4–5, 6
   and scintigraphy   79–89
prefrontal cortex (PFC)   6–8, 9
primary sclerosing cholangitis   71, 91, 155
primary sensory cortex (S1)   5–7
protoporphyrin IX (PPIX)   175–6
purified carbon   185, 190
push enteroscopy   217–24, 225

INDEX

radiation dose 99
radio frequency (RF) 144–5, 146, 148
Raman scattering 65
Raman spectroscopy 65
ratio fluorescence imaging (RFI) 62
reactive staining 182, 184–5, 188–9
reflux, scintigraphy/PET 81
Regula, J 179
resection 69, 70, 71, 72
　EASR 24, 27–8
　EATR 24, 26, 27–8
　EUS 43
　hepatocellular carcinoma 141
　LAER 23, 24, 25, 27–8
　metastases 146–8
　partial 142–3, 146–8
　wedge 23, 25, 27–8, 143
Riemann, J F 90–3
RO section 69, 72
robust estimation 200–4, 210
Rosch, T 43
Rust, G F 99

Scheffler, M 199
Schölmerich, J 158–70
Schomacker, K T 177
Schreyer, A G 194–8
Schubert, M 199
scintigraphy
　hepatobiliary 82
　and PET 79–89
　somatostatin receptor 86–8
screening
　colon cancer 102–3
　hepatocellular carcinoma 140
　liver cancer 145
　oesophageal cancers 183
　patient compliance 195
　virtual colonoscopy 97, 99
secondary somatosensory cortex (S2) 5–7
secretin test 47
secretin-enhanced MRCP 91
segmental TACE 144, 145
segmentectomy 143
sigmoidoscopy 53
　simulators 109, 110
Silverman, D H S 6
Silverman needle 16
Simbionix 110
simulators 53, 109–11
single-photon emission tomography (SPET) 4, 81, 86
small bowel
　cancer 55
　MRI 92
　pre-cancerous lesions 63
Smits, M E 37
SNOMED-DICOM microglossary 121, 123

somatostatin receptor scintigraphy 86–8
Sonazoid 134
sonography 83
　contrast ultrasound 163–4
　endosonography 40–9
　FNH 73
　percutaneous ultrasonography 90–1
Sonovist 132, 134
Sonovue 132
spasmolytic agents 98
specialized columnar epithelium (SCE) 186
sphincterotomy 109
spiral CT 43, 72, 162
splenomegaly 14, 129
squamous cell carcinoma 183, 186
squamous epithelium 226–7
Stael von Holstein, C S 176, 177
steatosis 17
stenting 28, 33, 34
　EUS 42
　MPD strictures 36–8
stereo endoscopes 199–200
stimulated acoustic enhancement (SAE), microbubbles 134
stomach
　cancer 55, 189
　chromoendoscopy 188
　laparoscopy and endoscopy 27
　LIFE-GI 62
stroke 9
structure from motion problem 199, 200
supplementary motor cortex 6
surface nodularity 127–8, 130
surface rendering 96–7

T1 carcinoma 55–6
Taylor-Robinson, S D 132–9
texturing 206
thalamus 6–7
thermal ablation procedures 148
Thiis-Evensen, E 102
Thompson, D G 4
thoracotomy 27
Thormählen, T 199–211
three-dimensional coordinates calculation 204–5
three-dimensional endoscopy 199–211
three-dimensional imaging 94–106
three-dimensional reconstruction 204–6
Tio, T L 42, 43
tissue staining see chromoendoscopy
toluidine blue 184, 186
training models 109–11
transarterial chemoembolization (TACE) 141, 143–4
　segmental 144, 145
transarterial embolization (TAE) 143–4
transplants, liver 71, 141, 142, 146

234

INDEX

Treichel, U 13–20
triangle mesh generation 205–6
tuberculosis 14
tumours
  see also individual types
  cholangiocarcinoma 42
  early detection 55–68
  fluorescence endoscopy 173–81
  gallbladder 154
  laparoscopy and endoscopy 27, 28
  oesophagus 27
  pancreatic cancer 42–4
  PET 83–6
  preoperative imaging 69–75
Tytgat, G N J 43

ulcerative colitis 60, 66, 173
  cancer 56
  fluorescence endoscopy 178, 179
  PDT 59
ulcerative pancolitis 179
ultrasound
  see also endoscopic ultrasound (EUS)
  biliary disease 151–7
  contrast agents 132–9
  diffuse liver disease 127–31
  interventional therapy 140–50
  intraductal 42, 155–6
  unclear liver tumours 158–70

Verres needle 15
video capsule 63
video endoscopy 53

video push enteroscopy 225
videolaparoscopy 22
Vining, D J 194
virtual colonography, CT- or MRI-based 194–8
virtual colonoscopy 92, 97–103
virtual endoscopy 100
virtual gastroscopy 196
virtual pathology 196
vital staining 182–3, 184
Vo-Dinh, T 177
Vogl, T J 148
volume rendering 97
volumetry, liver 70

Wagner, S 151–7
Wallace, M B 46
wedge resection 23, 25, 27–8, 143
Wiersema, M J 45
Wietek, B 3–12
wireless capsule endoscopy 215–24, 225
Wong, K 96
World Organization of Digestive Endoscopy (OMED) 113, 115, 123

Yasuda, K 42
Yeung, S Y 200

'Z' line 226
Zeeh, J M 13–20
Zimmerman, M J 46
zoom endoscopy 56, 62–4
Zuccarro, 47

Falk Symposium Series

43. Reutter W, Popper H, Arias IM, Heinrich PC, Keppler D, Landmann L, eds.: *Modulation of Liver Cell Expression*. Falk Symposium No. 43. 1987   ISBN: 0-85200-677-2*
44. Boyer JL, Bianchi L, eds.: *Liver Cirrhosis*. Falk Symposium No. 44. 1987
    ISBN: 0-85200-993-3*
45. Paumgartner G, Stiehl A, Gerok W, eds.: *Bile Acids and the Liver*. Falk Symposium No. 45. 1987   ISBN: 0-85200-675-6*
46. Goebell H, Peskar BM, Malchow H, eds.: *Inflammatory Bowel Diseases – Basic Research & Clinical Implications*. Falk Symposium No. 46. 1988   ISBN: 0-7462-0067-6*
47. Bianchi L, Holt P, James OFW, Butler RN, eds.: *Aging in Liver and Gastrointestinal Tract*. Falk Symposium No. 47. 1988   ISBN: 0-7462-0066-8*
48. Heilmann C, ed.: *Calcium-Dependent Processes in the Liver*. Falk Symposium No. 48. 1988   ISBN: 0-7462-0075-7*
50. Singer MV, Goebell H, eds.: *Nerves and the Gastrointestinal Tract*. Falk Symposium No. 50. 1989   ISBN: 0-7462-0114-1
51. Bannasch P, Keppler D, Weber G, eds.: *Liver Cell Carcinoma*. Falk Symposium No. 51. 1989   ISBN: 0-7462-0111-7
52. Paumgartner G, Stiehl A, Gerok W, eds.: *Trends in Bile Acid Research*. Falk Symposium No. 52. 1989   ISBN: 0-7462-0112-5
53. Paumgartner G, Stiehl A, Barbara L, Roda E, eds.: *Strategies for the Treatment of Hepatobiliary Diseases*. Falk Symposium No. 53. 1990   ISBN: 0-7923-8903-4
54. Bianchi L, Gerok W, Maier K-P, Deinhardt F, eds.: *Infectious Diseases of the Liver*. Falk Symposium No. 54. 1990   ISBN: 0-7923-8902-6
55. Falk Symposium No. 55 not published
55B. Hadziselimovic F, Herzog B, Bürgin-Wolff A, eds.: *Inflammatory Bowel Disease and Coeliac Disease in Children*. International Falk Symposium. 1990 ISBN 0-7462-0125-7
56. Williams CN, eds.: *Trends in Inflammatory Bowel Disease Therapy*. Falk Symposium No. 56. 1990   ISBN: 0-7923-8952-2
57. Bock KW, Gerok W, Matern S, Schmid R, eds.: *Hepatic Metabolism and Disposition of Endo- and Xenobiotics*. Falk Symposium No. 57. 1991   ISBN: 0-7923-8953-0
58. Paumgartner G, Stiehl A, Gerok W, eds.: *Bile Acids as Therapeutic Agents: From Basic Science to Clinical Practice*. Falk Symposium No. 58. 1991   ISBN: 0-7923-8954-9
59. Halter F, Garner A, Tytgat GNJ, eds.: *Mechanisms of Peptic Ulcer Healing*. Falk Symposium No. 59. 1991   ISBN: 0-7923-8955-7
60. Goebell H, Ewe K, Malchow H, Koelbel Ch, eds.: *Inflammatory Bowel Diseases – Progress in Basic Research and Clinical Implications*. Falk Symposium No. 60. 1991
    ISBN: 0-7923-8956-5
61. Falk Symposium No. 61 not published
62. Dowling RH, Folsch UR, Löser Ch, eds.: *Polyamines in the Gastrointestinal Tract*. Falk Symposium No. 62. 1992   ISBN: 0-7923-8976-X
63. Lentze MJ, Reichen J, eds.: *Paediatric Cholestasis: Novel Approaches to Treatment*. Falk Symposium No. 63. 1992   ISBN: 0-7923-8977-8
64. Demling L, Frühmorgen P, eds.: *Non-Neoplastic Diseases of the Anorectum*. Falk Symposium No. 64. 1992   ISBN: 0-7923-8979-4
64B. Gressner AM, Ramadori G, eds.: *Molecular and Cell Biology of Liver Fibrogenesis*. International Falk Symposium. 1992   ISBN: 0-7923-8980-8

*These titles were published under the MTP Press imprint.

Falk Symposium Series

65. Hadziselimovic F, Herzog B, eds.: *Inflammatory Bowel Diseases and Morbus Hirschprung.* Falk Symposium No. 65. 1992   ISBN: 0-7923-8995-6
66. Martin F, McLeod RS, Sutherland LR, Williams CN, eds.: *Trends in Inflammatory Bowel Disease Therapy.* Falk Symposium No. 66. 1993   ISBN: 0-7923-8827-5
67. Schölmerich J, Kruis W, Goebell H, Hohenberger W, Gross V, eds.: *Inflammatory Bowel Diseases – Pathophysiology as Basis of Treatment.* Falk Symposium No. 67. 1993
ISBN: 0-7923-8996-4
68. Paumgartner G, Stiehl A, Gerok W, eds.: *Bile Acids and The Hepatobiliary System: From Basic Science to Clinical Practice.* Falk Symposium No. 68. 1993
ISBN: 0-7923-8829-1
69. Schmid R, Bianchi L, Gerok W, Maier K-P, eds.: *Extrahepatic Manifestations in Liver Diseases.* Falk Symposium No. 69. 1993   ISBN: 0-7923-8821-6
70. Meyer zum Büschenfelde K-H, Hoofnagle J, Manns M, eds.: *Immunology and Liver.* Falk Symposium No. 70. 1993   ISBN: 0-7923-8830-5
71. Surrenti C, Casini A, Milani S, Pinzani M , eds.: *Fat-Storing Cells and Liver Fibrosis.* Falk Symposium No. 71. 1994   ISBN: 0-7923-8842-9
72. Rachmilewitz D, ed.: *Inflammatory Bowel Diseases – 1994.* Falk Symposium No. 72. 1994   ISBN: 0-7923-8845-3
73. Binder HJ, Cummings J, Soergel KH, eds.: *Short Chain Fatty Acids.* Falk Symposium No. 73. 1994   ISBN: 0-7923-8849-6
73B. Möllmann HW, May B, eds.: *Glucocorticoid Therapy in Chronic Inflammatory Bowel Disease: from basic principles to rational therapy.* International Falk Workshop. 1996
ISBN 0-7923-8708-2
74. Keppler D, Jungermann K, eds.: *Transport in the Liver.* Falk Symposium No. 74. 1994
ISBN: 0-7923-8858-5
74B. Stange EF, ed.: *Chronic Inflammatory Bowel Disease.* Falk Symposium. 1995
ISBN: 0-7923-8876-3
75. van Berge Henegouwen GP, van Hoek B, De Groote J, Matern S, Stockbrügger RW, eds.: *Cholestatic Liver Diseases: New Strategies for Prevention and Treatment of Hepatobiliary and Cholestatic Liver Diseases.* Falk Symposium 75. 1994.
ISBN: 0-7923-8867-4
76. Monteiro E, Tavarela Veloso F, eds.: *Inflammatory Bowel Diseases: New Insights into Mechanisms of Inflammation and Challenges in Diagnosis and Treatment.* Falk Symposium 76. 1995.   ISBN 0-7923-8884-4
77. Singer MV, Ziegler R, Rohr G, eds.: *Gastrointestinal Tract and Endocrine System.* Falk Symposium 77. 1995.   ISBN 0-7923-8877-1
78. Decker K, Gerok W, Andus T, Gross V, eds.: *Cytokines and the Liver.* Falk Symposium 78. 1995.   ISBN 0-7923-8878-X
79. Holstege A, Schölmerich J, Hahn EG, eds.: *Portal Hypertension.* Falk Symposium 79. 1995.   ISBN 0-7923-8879-8
80. Hofmann AF, Paumgartner G, Stiehl A, eds.: *Bile Acids in Gastroenterology: Basic and Clinical Aspects.* Falk Symposium 80. 1995   ISBN 0-7923-8880-1
81. Riecken EO, Stallmach A, Zeitz M, Heise W, eds.: *Malignancy and Chronic Inflammation in the Gastrointestinal Tract – New Concepts.* Falk Symposium 81. 1995
ISBN 0-7923-8889-5
82. Fleig WE, ed.: *Inflammatory Bowel Diseases: New Developments and Standards.* Falk Symposium 82. 1995   ISBN 0-7923-8890-6

Falk Symposium Series

82B. Paumgartner G, Beuers U, eds.: *Bile Acids in Liver Diseases.* International Falk Workshop. 1995   ISBN 0-7923-8891-7

83. Dobrilla G, Felder M, de Pretis G, eds.: *Advances in Hepatobiliary and Pancreatic Diseases: Special Clinical Topics.* Falk Symposium 83. 1995.   ISBN 0-7923-8892-5

84. Fromm H, Leuschner U, eds.: *Bile Acids – Cholestasis – Gallstones: Advances in Basic and Clinical Bile Acid Research.* Falk Symposium 84. 1995   ISBN 0-7923-8893-3

85. Tytgat GNJ, Bartelsman JFWM, van Deventer SJH, eds.: *Inflammatory Bowel Diseases.* Falk Symposium 85. 1995   ISBN 0-7923-8894-1

86. Berg PA, Leuschner U, eds.: *Bile Acids and Immunology.* Falk Symposium 86. 1996   ISBN 0-7923-8700-7

87. Schmid R, Bianchi L, Blum HE, Gerok W, Maier KP, Stalder GA, eds.: *Acute and Chronic Liver Diseases: Molecular Biology and Clinics.* Falk Symposium 87. 1996   ISBN 0-7923-8701-5

88. Blum HE, Wu GY, Wu CH, eds.: *Molecular Diagnosis and Gene Therapy.* Falk Symposium 88. 1996   ISBN 0-7923-8702-3

88B. Poupon RE, Reichen J, eds.: *Surrogate Markers to Assess Efficacy of TReatment in Chronic Liver Diseases.* International Falk Workshop. 1996   ISBN 0-7923-8705-8

89. Reyes HB, Leuschner U, Arias IM, eds.: *Pregnancy, Sex Hormones and the Liver.* Falk Symposium 89. 1996   ISBN 0-7923-8704-X

89B. Broelsch CE, Burdelski M, Rogiers X, eds.: *Cholestatic Liver Diseases in Children and Adults.* International Falk Workshop. 1996   ISBN 0-7923-8710-4

90. Lam S-K, Paumgartner P, Wang B, eds.: *Update on Hepatobiliary Diseases 1996.* Falk Symposium 90. 1996   ISBN 0-7923-8715-5

91. Hadziselimovic F, Herzog B, eds.: *Inflammatory Bowel Diseases and Chronic Recurrent Abdominal Pain.* Falk Symposium 91. 1996   ISBN 0-7923-8722-8

91B. Alvaro D, Benedetti A, Strazzabosco M, eds.: *Vanishing Bile Duct Syndrome – Pathophysiology and Treatment.* International Falk Workshop. 1996   ISBN 0-7923-8721-X

92. Gerok W, Loginov AS, Pokrowskij VI, eds.: *New Trends in Hepatology 1996.* Falk Symposium 92. 1997   ISBN 0-7923-8723-6

93. Paumgartner G, Stiehl A, Gerok W, eds.: *Bile Acids in Hepatobiliary Diseases – Basic Research and Clinical Application.* Falk Symposium 93. 1997   ISBN 0-7923-8725-2

94. Halter F, Winton D, Wright NA, eds.: *The Gut as a Model in Cell and Molecular Biology.* Falk Symposium 94. 1997   ISBN 0-7923-8726-0

94B. Kruse-Jarres JD, Schölmerich J, eds.: *Zinc and Diseases of the Digestive Tract.* International Falk Workshop. 1997   ISBN 0-7923-8724-4

95. Ewe K, Eckardt VF, Enck P, eds.: *Constipation and Anorectal Insufficiency.* Falk Symposium 95. 1997   ISBN 0-7923-8727-9

96. Andus T, Goebell H, Layer P, Schölmerich J, eds.: *Inflammatory Bowel Disease – from Bench to Bedside.* Falk Symposium 96. 1997   ISBN 0-7923-8728-7

97. Campieri M, Bianchi-Porro G, Fiocchi C, Schölmerich J, eds. *Clinical Challenges in Inflammatory Bowel Diseases: Diagnosis, Prognosis and Treatment.* Falk Symposium 97. 1998   ISBN 0-7923-8733-3

98. Lembcke B, Kruis W, Sartor RB, eds. *Systemic Manifestations of IBD: The Pending Challenge for Subtle Diagnosis and Treatment.* Falk Symposium 98. 1998   ISBN 0-7923-8734-1

Falk Symposium Series

99. Goebell H, Holtmann G, Talley NJ, eds. *Functional Dyspepsia and Irritable Bowel Syndrome: Concepts and Controversies.* Falk Symposium 99. 1998
ISBN 0-7923-8735-X
100. Blum HE, Bode Ch, Bode JCh, Sartor RB, eds. *Gut and the Liver.* Falk Symposium 100. 1998
ISBN 0-7923-8736-8
101. Rachmilewitz D, ed. *V International Symposium on Inflammatory Bowel Diseases.* Falk Symposium 101. 1998
ISBN 0-7923-8743-0
102. Manns MP, Boyer JL, Jansen PLM, Reichen J, eds. *Cholestatic Liver Diseases.* Falk Symposium 102. 1998
ISBN 0-7923-8746-5
102B. Manns MP, Chapman RW, Stiehl A, Wiesner R, eds. *Primary Sclerosing Cholangitis.* International Falk Workshop. 1998.
ISBN 0-7923-8745-7
103. Häussinger D, Jungermann K, eds. *Liver and Nervous System.* Falk Symposium 102. 1998
ISBN 0-7924-8742-2
103B. Häussinger D, Heinrich PC, eds. *Signalling in the Liver.* International Falk Workshop. 1998
ISBN 0-7923-8744-9
103C. Fleig W, ed. *Normal and Malignant Liver Cell Growth.* International Falk Workshop. 1998
ISBN 0-7923-8748-1
104. Stallmach A, Zeitz M, Strober W, MacDonald TT, Lochs H, eds. *Induction and Modulation of Gastrointestinal Inflammation.* Falk Symposium 104. 1998
ISBN 0-7923-8747-3
105. Emmrich J, Liebe S, Stange EF, eds. *Innovative Concepts in Inflammatory Bowel Diseases.* Falk Symposium 105. 1999
ISBN 0-7923-8749-X
106. Rutgeerts P, Colombel J-F, Hanauer SB, Schölmerich J, Tytgat GNJ, van Gossum A, eds. *Advances in Inflammatory Bowel Diseases.* Falk Symposium 106. 1999
ISBN 0-7923-8750-3
107. Špičák J, Boyer J, Gilat T, Kotrlik K, Mareček Z, Paumgartner G, eds. *Diseases of the Liver and the Bile Ducts – New Aspects and Clinical Implications.* Falk Symposium 107. 1999
ISBN 0-7923-8751-1
108. Paumgartner G, Stiehl A, Gerok W, Keppler D, Leuschner U, eds. *Bile Acids and Cholestasis.* Falk Symposium 108. 1999
ISBN 0-7923-8752-X
109. Schmiegel W, Schölmerich J, eds. *Colorectal Cancer – Molecular Mechanisms, Premalignant State and its Prevention.* Falk Symposium 109. 1999
ISBN 0-7923-8753-8
110. Domschke W, Stoll R, Brasitus TA, Kagnoff MF, eds. *Intestinal Mucosa and its Diseases – Pathophysiology and Clinics.* Falk Symposium 110. 1999
ISBN 0-7923-8754-6
110B. Northfield TC, Ahmed HA, Jazwari RP, Zentler-Munro PL, eds. *Bile Acids in Hepatobiliary Disease.* Falk Workshop. 2000
ISBN 0-7923-8755-4
111. Rogler G, Kullmann F, Rutgeerts P, Sartor RB, Schölmerich J, eds. *IBD at the End of its First Century.* Falk Symposium 111. 2000
ISBN 0-7923-8756-2
112. Krammer HJ, Singer MV, eds. *Neurogastroenterology: From the Basics to the Clinics.* Falk Symposium 112. 2000
ISBN 0-7923-8757-0
113. Andus T, Rogler G, Schlottmann K, Frick E, Adler G, Schmiegel W, Zeitz M, Schölmerich J, eds. *Cytokines and Cell Homeostasis in the Gastrointestinal Tract.* Falk Symposium 113. 2000
ISBN 0-7923-8758-9
114. Manns MP, Paumgartner G, Leuschner U, eds. *Immunology and Liver.* Falk Symposium 114. 2000
ISBN 0-7923-8759-7

Falk Symposium Series

115. Boyer JL, Blum HE, Maier K-P, Sauerbruch T, Stalder GA, eds. *Liver Cirrhosis and its Development.* Falk Symposium 115. 2000 ISBN 0-7923-8760-0
116. Riemann JF, Neuhaus H, eds. *Interventional Endoscopy in Hepatology.* Falk Symposium 116. 2000 ISBN 0-7923-8761-9
116A. Dienes HP, Schirmacher P, Brechot C, Okuda K, eds. *Chronic Hepatitis: New Concepts of Pathogenesis, Diagnosis and Treatment.* Falk Workshop. 2000
ISBN 0-7923-8763-5
117. Gerbes AL, Beuers U, Jüngst D, Pape GR, Sackmann M, Sauerbruch T, eds. *Hepatology 2000 – Symposium in Honour of Gustav Paumgartner.* Falk Symposium 117. 2000
ISBN 0-7923-8765-1
117A. Acalovschi M, Paumgartner G, eds. *Hepatobiliary Diseases: Cholestasis and Gallstones.* Falk Workshop. 2000 ISBN 0-7923-8770-8
118. Frühmorgen P, Bruch H-P, eds. *Non-Neoplastic Diseases of the Anorectum.* Falk Symposium 118. 2001 ISBN 0-7923-8766-X
119. Fellermann K, Jewell DP, Sandborn WJ, Schölmerich J, Stange EF, eds. *Immunosuppression in Inflammatory Bowel Diseases – Standards, New Developments, Future Trends.* Falk Symposium 119. 2001 ISBN 0-7923-8767-8
120. van Berge Henegouwen GP, Keppler D, Leuschner U, Paumgartner G, Stiehl A, eds. *Biology of Bile Acids in Health and Disease.* Falk Symposium 120. 2001
ISBN 0-7923-8768-6
121. Leuschner U, James OFW, Dancygier H, eds. *Steatohepatitis (NASH and ASH).* Falk Symposium 121. 2001 ISBN 0-7923-8769-4
121A. Matern S, Boyer JL, Keppler D, Meier-Abt PJ, eds. *Hepatobiliary Transport: From Bench to Bedside.* Falk Workshop. 2001 ISBN 0-7923-8771-6
122. Campieri M, Fiocchi C, Hanauer SB, Jewell DP, Rachmilewitz R, Schölmerich J, eds. *Inflammatory Bowel Disease – A Clinical Case Approach to Pathophysiology, Diagnosis, and Treatment.* Falk Symposium 122. 2002 ISBN 0-7923-8772-4
123. Rachmilewitz D, Modigliani R, Podolsky DK, Sachar DB, Tozun N, eds. *VI International Symposium on Inflammatory Bowel Diseases.* Falk Symposium 123. 2002
ISBN 0-7923-8773-2
124. Hagenmüller F, Manns MP, Musmann H-G, Riemann JF, eds. *Medical Imaging in Gastroenterology and Hepatology.* Falk Symposium 124. 2002 ISBN 0-7923-8774-0
125. Gressner AM, Heinrich PC, Matern S, eds. *Cytokines in Liver Injury and Repair.* Falk Symposium 125. 2002 ISBN 0-7923-8775-9
126. Gupta S, Jansen PLM, Klempnauer J, Manns MP, eds. *Hepatocyte Transplantation.* Falk Symposium 126. 2002 ISBN 0-7923-8776-7
127. Hadziselimovic F, ed. *Autoimmune Diseases in Paediatric Gastroenterology.* Falk Symposium 127. 2002 ISBN 0-7923-8778-3
127A. Berr F, Bruix J, Hauss J, Wands J, Wittekind Ch, eds. *Malignant Liver Tumours: Basic Concepts and Clinical Management.* Falk Workshop. 2002 ISBN 0-7923-8779-1